there's A Vegan in the Kitchen:

Viva la Vegan's Easy & tasty Plant-Based Recipes.

Book Details

Epicentre Equilibrium Publishing

Copyright © 2013 by Leigh-Chantelle
Food Photography & Author Portrait by Carol Slater Photography (c-s-p.com.au)
Cover & Illustrations by Sarah Kiser (artbysarahkiser.com)
Food Styling by Leigh-Chantelle, Carol Slater and Gwen Koch
All Recipes © Leigh-Chantelle & Viva la Vegan!
Lettering by Leigh-Chantelle (leigh-chantelle.com)
Design by Bambi Wants Revenge (bambiwantsrevenge.com)
All rights reserved
ISBN 978-0-9808484-4-1
www.epicentreequilibrium.com

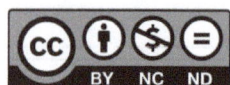

About the Book

'There's a Vegan in the Kitchen: Viva la Vegan's Easy and Tasty Plant-Based Recipes' the book, started after I graduated from my Naturopathy and Nutrition studies in 2005 and I decided to release my first recipe calendar to show people how to heal themselves with food. Three recipe calendars were released in 2006, 2007 and 2008, then later becoming recycled recipe cards.

'There's a Vegan in the Kitchen' includes 36 of my original vegan recipes that are all nutritionally balanced, healthful and easy to prepare. These are delicious alternatives for meat-free, dairy-free, egg-free eating, with a large amount of the recipes also wheat- and gluten-free. See the gluten-free, soy-free and nut-free icons on each recipe page. There are full-colour photographs for each recipe, inspirational quotes and information, combined with wonderful illustrations by Sarah Kiser.

These meals have been made countless times for gatherings, dinner parties, potlucks and more. People always ask me, "What do you eat?" I can say that since becoming vegan in early 1997, that I have discovered so many more grains, nuts, seeds and vegetables than I ever thought existed!

When using this book, please be creative as much as possible with your own version of the recipes. Add and subtract what you will to suit your own tastebuds. Always experiment with your cooking and search for new ingredients. Frequent Chinese, Indian and other stores that cater predominately to another culture than your own. This will open up the variety of foods that you consume so that you never become bored with your diet. Buy fresh, organic produce as much as you can and support locally owned, family-run businesses. Think locally to act globally.

A low fat, wholefoods, varied vegan diet is easy to follow, great for your health, the health of our planet and doesn't harm any of our animal friends. I hope this book inspires you to take control of your health and lead by example to promote a compassionate lifestyle to all whom you encounter.

Please see my website, vivalavegan.net for more information on becoming part of the vegan revolution.

True peace begins on your plate,

Leigh-Chantelle

Contents

the History of Viva la Vegan!

In September 2005, I graduated from the Australian Institute of Applied Science in Stones Corner, Brisbane, Australia; where I had completed my Advanced Diploma in Naturopathy, Advanced Diploma in Nutrition and Advanced Diploma in Western Herbal Medicine.

I remember my favourite lecturer and friend, Mark Nicholson had said to us over and over again that only one in twenty students who graduate would actually go on to practice. I believed I would be that one who would practice.

My passion had always been vegan and vegetarian health – this was why I had decided to study Nutrition in the first place. However when I got to the end of my three years studying I didn't want to open my own business and didn't want to work in a health food store, so I ended up going back to my first love: music (retail.) I had always wanted to release a recipe book and I thought that would be a huge undertaking, so I decided to use my skills and release a recipe calendar first, as twelve recipes should be quite easy to compile.

I have an exercise book full of all my recipes, which I've had for years. Each time I create a new meal, I make sure to take a photo of the dish and write down the ingredients and the method of preparation and cooking. My first task in creating the calendar was to go through the recipes I already had, add some new ones if needed and compile them all together. My sister, Louise and I went to the local park to my yoga spot, where she took some photos with a meal I had cooked the night before. These would be the photos for the covers of my 2006 calendar.

Next I needed to find someone who could design the calendar for me. I always know exactly how I want things to look, but I need someone to actually put my vision into reality. A friend of Lou's was studying a graphic design class at TAFE (Training And Further Education) with another guy, Ziggy who became my go-to guy for all things design. Ziggy and I worked together for two years developing the calendar and learning from each other.

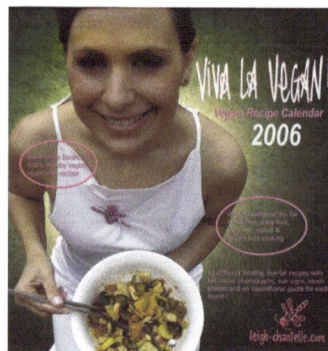

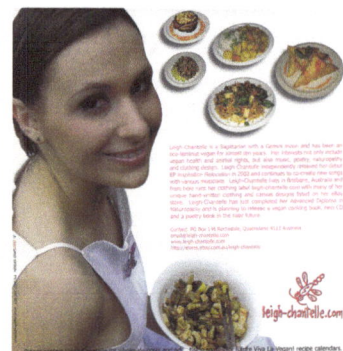

The first Viva la Vegan! Recipe Calendar was released at the end of 2005 and promoted on my leigh-chantelle.com website and at various interstate vegan events. The aim was to get local businesses to advertise in the calendar, but as I only had a short amount of time in between leaving college and the release of the calendar, it didn't happen as planned. I met some great people and even had a request to join as a chef in Brisbane's only (at the time) vegan restaurant, The Forest. However, I had just signed up to work at JB Hi-Fi as a music consultant.

Preparation for my second calendar in 2006 began my experimenting with alternative (at the time) grains. This was inspired by two of my friends who lent me amazing books that began my search for alternative ingredients. Melissa from college lent me 'Allergy Cooking with Ease' by Nicolette M Dumke and Benjamin from school lent me 'Vegan on a Shoestring' by the People's Potato Collective. Another inspiration was 'The Great American Detox Diet' by (then-vegan) Alex Jamieson, a book that encourages people to heal themselves with food, as I also promote.

The alternative grains I learned about have been around for centuries from ancient cultures in various parts of the world. I prefer to cook without wheat-based ingredients most of the time – it's better for you and this also means that everyone will be able to eat your meals.

My favourite alternative grain (really a seed) at the time was – and still is – quinoa (pronounced keen-wa.) It's a complete protein, meaning that it has all of the building blocks of protein, known as amino acids, in one place. There's also amaranth, barley, brown rice, buckwheat, cornmeal (polenta), kamut, millet, oats, rye, spelt and wild rice. Most of these grains can be cooked with the ratio of 1:2 grains to water.

Sometime in 2006, I launched the vivalavegan.net website to answer the fast-growing interest in veganism, and various requests from other vegans to share recipes, articles and more. Ziggy's friend, Simon from Studio Lucid created the original website for me:

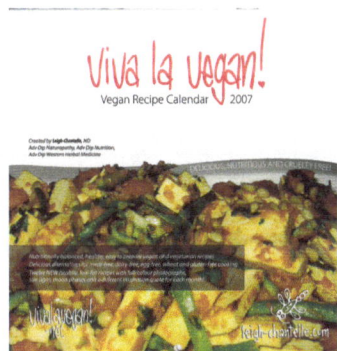

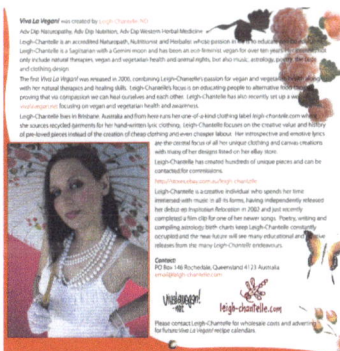

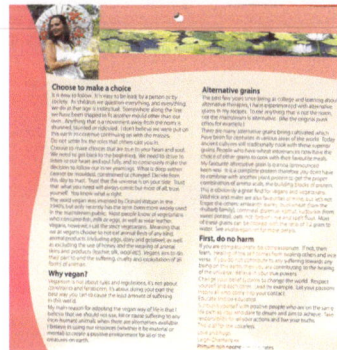

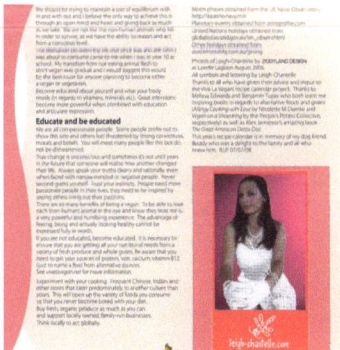

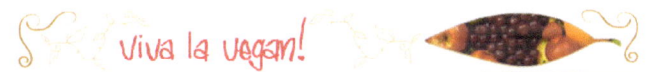

Photos for the upcoming 2007 calendar were taken by Ziggy in August 2006 at Lavelle Lagoon, Greenbank. I dedicated the calendar to my family's dog friend, Buddy who had passed over on the 7 July.

I decided that the 2008 calendars would be my last due to the short shelf life of calendars, usually only October – January. My focus was instead on building up my website to create more of an interactive online space for vegans. We added an audio-visual section, forum, member's section, vegan merchandise and advertising. Simon continued with the website updates and re-designs until 2009 when I also released my Detox Diet eBook.

Simon also took over the design for the third calendar and we started using the colour red, which is more suited to food. Along with the full-colour photographs for each recipe and the inspirational quotes, I also added some food facts. The black and white photographs for the 2008 calendar were taken by photographer and friend, Hamish Cairns in September 2007 at Southport.

While I was working at JB Hi-Fi I made a lot of wonderful friends, most of whose eating habits were atrocious. I remember one day at work one of my colleagues mentioned that he eats fast food for every meal and I was incredibly shocked. I still am shocked that people regularly eat rubbish all the time, which they pass off as food – for themselves and their families.

I decided that the 2008 calendar was going to be filled with healthier vegan versions of the meals that so many of my friends loved to eat. This became an important focus for me with a lot of the meals I've created since - converting non-vegan foods that my friends like into more healthier versions. These meals were still great tasting, environmentally sustainable and just as importantly, not harmful to any of our animal friends.

I made a lot of friends and began my vegan networking during the course of the years of releasing my vegan recipe calendars. When I first became vegan in early 1997 it was a lot harder to find vegan products. The supermarket stocked one brand of soymilk, if you were lucky. Every now and then you would be excited to find dark chocolate or even carob chocolate at a health food store.

Nowadays everything you can think of has a vegan alternative. My local supermarket and health food store both have a lot of vegan products, plus there are so many online vegan stores and vegan restaurants now. Most major cities (including Brisbane where I live) have vegan storefronts. To me, being vegan is mighty easy.

My website was relaunched and re-designed in June 2010 by Sharon and Terry from Design Voodoo. It has grown in so many ways and finally after many incarnations, in 2013 it is where I always aimed it to be. It now has regular (mostly daily) content including videos, articles from various authors, blogs, interviews, various eBooks, print books, coaching, more advertisers and even an affiliate section. The addition of the majority of these sections is due to feedback over the years, including the search bar.

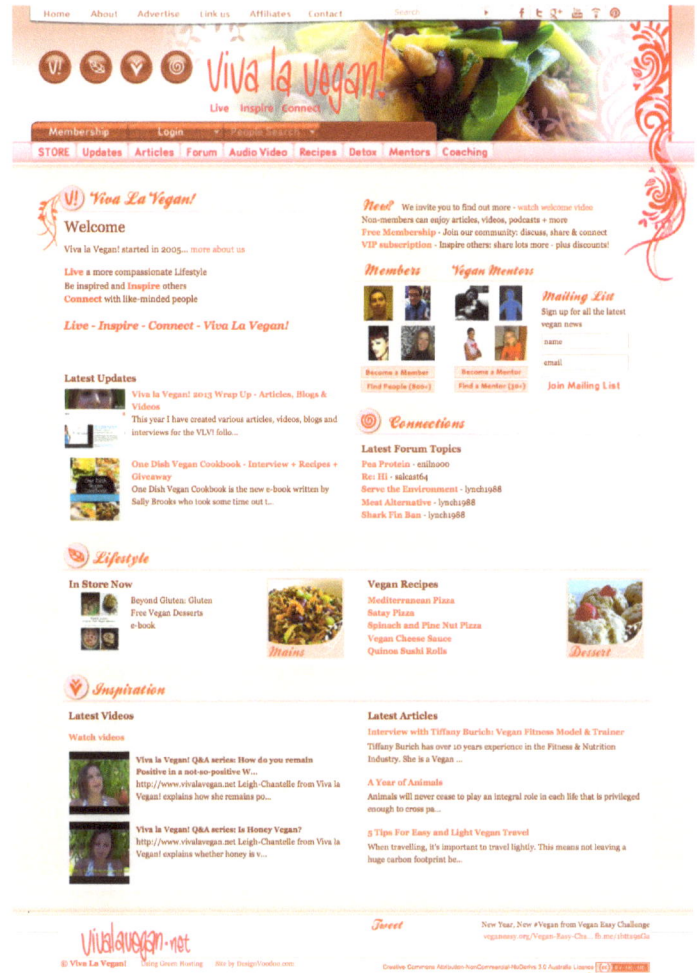

The remaining calendars were cut up, the recipes glued back to back, laminated together, hole-punched at the tops and tied together for sale and donations to animal sanctuaries. I no longer have any of these calendars or recycled recipe cards.

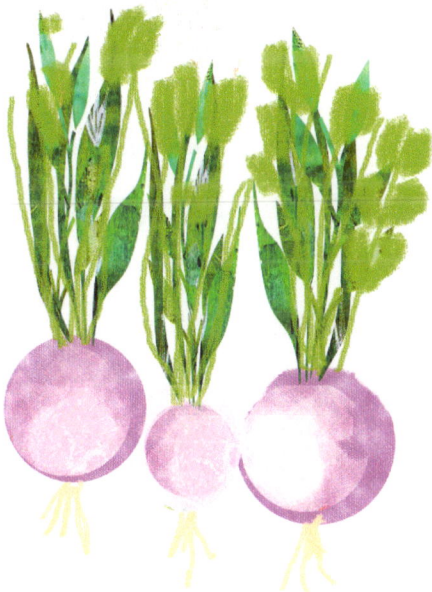

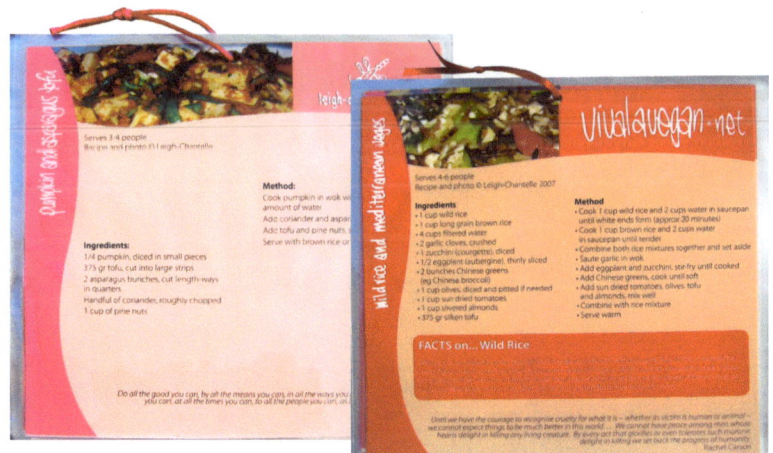

Early in 2013 I decided to put a book together with all of the recipes from the three calendars.

Sometime in early 2013, my friend and go-to designer, Adele and I were working on the upcoming collection of my recipe calendars into book format. The photos would have to be redone and a better name than 'The Viva la Vegan! Recipe Calendar Collection' was needed. My friend and photographer, Carol and I spent three days shooting the photos for this book over a couple of weeks and I spent about a week with the food preparation.

A vegan artist friend of mine from FaceBook, Sarah had mentioned online that she had always wanted to illustrate a vegan recipe book. I sent her an email to see if she was interested in working on this project with me - you can see her wonderful illustrations throughout the book. The three vegan gals mentioned and I created this recipe book together. We are all committed to our art and the vegan cause. I do hope you enjoy it.

Viva la Vegan! is on just about every social media channel you can think of: FaceBook, Google+, iTunes for our podcasts, Pinterest, Twitter and YouTube. There is more and more interest in a vegan diet and the vegan lifestyle each year, and it will only grow stronger. I'm grateful and humbled that vivalavegan. net and our social media channels are where a large majority of vegans and the vegan-curious get their regular positive vegan information.

Thank you to all who have given their advice and imput to the Viva la Vegan! recipe calendar project and website since 2005. In particular, my vegan friends from all over the world - from MySpace, Twitter, FaceBook and various animal liberation, animal rights, vegetarian and vegan groups.

Also thank you to the Viva la Vegan! fans and followers on FaceBook, Google+, iTunes, MySpace, Pinterest, Twitter and YouTube, who remind me that the vegan community is alive, strong and healthy all over our world.

Always believe in the power of positive influence and the most important power of all, which comes from YOU.

Leigh-Chantelle

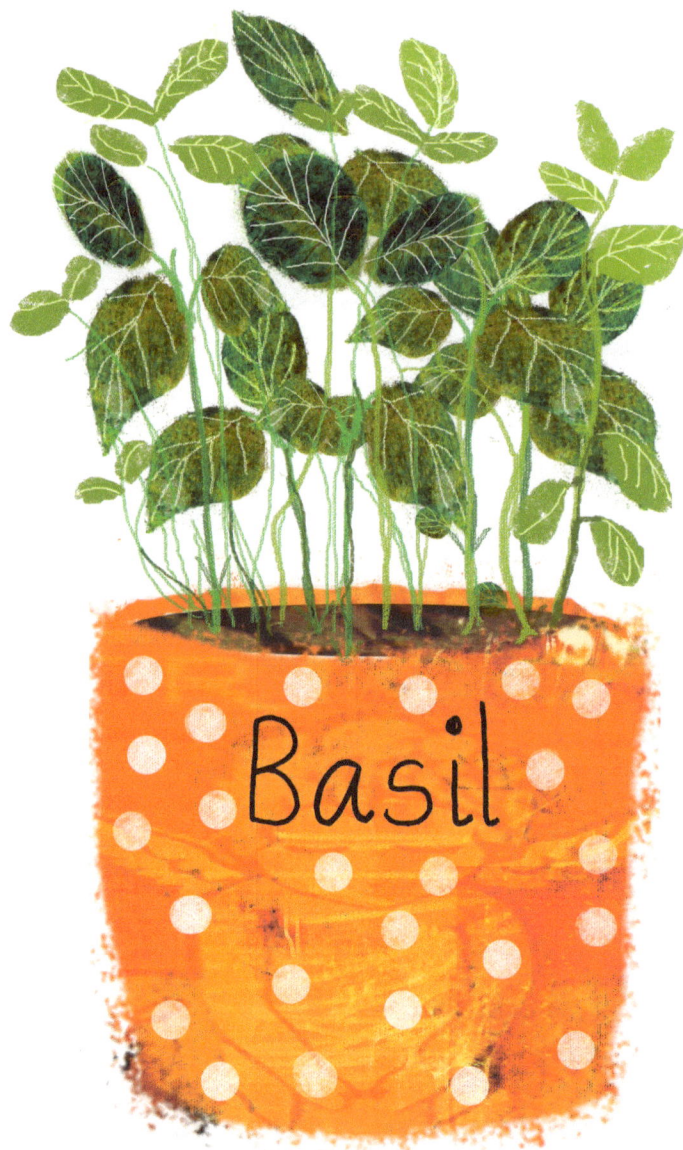

Basil

SINCERE GRATITUDE TO THE FOLLOWING PEOPLE:

Ziggy from ZD Creative Solutions
zdcreativesolutions.com
For designing the first two calendars and taking the photos for the second calendar.

Simon from Studio Lucid
studiolucid.net
For designing the last calendar and the first incarnation of my vivalavegan.net website.

Louise Koch
For her photography on the first calendar and various help over the years.

Hamish Cairns
hamishcairns.com
For his wonderful photography for my last calendar.

Michelle Jones
For coming up with the original name for the calendars, which would also become the website name.

My Mum, Gwen & Dad, Bill
For their countless help over the years with all my projects - both big and small.

Loren Lebke
Who gave me my first magazine cover (with a photo by Lou) for the then 'New Vegetarian and Natural Health' magazine Autumn 2006 edition. She says she made me, so who am I to argue!

The ladies from Eve's clinic
Who gave me constant encouragement for this project in 2005 when we were just about to graduate college.

Melissa Edwards
For lending me the 'Allergy Cooking with Ease' book by Nicolette M Dumke.

Benjamin Tupas
For lending me the 'Vegan on a Shoestring' book by the People's Potato Collective.

My JB work friends
Who offered their advice, taste testing and encouragement, as well as letting me read every label and ingredients list they ever had.

Sharon and Terry from Design Voodoo
designvoodoo.com
For my various websites, design and advice since 2010.

Carol Slater
c-s-p.com.au
For the wonderful food photography and helping with styling – we've become quite the food stylists.

Adele Walker
bambiwantsrevenge.com
For her always amazing graphic design, plus pushing me to get professional photos and a better title.

Sarah Kiser
artbysarahkiser.com
For her remarkable renditions of the ingredients and utensils list into illustrations – plus the fantastic cover.

Paul Mahony
terrastendo.net
For his help with compiling the environmental information.

Jack Norris, RD
jacknorrisrd.com
For his help with updating the health information.

Jim Campbell
The winner of the name this book competition – and to all of the people who voted for it online.

Why Vegan?

There are many reasons why someone would choose to become vegan.

I decided to become vegan just after I finished high school in early 1997. I realised the dairy products and eggs that I was consuming every now and then were causing just as much, if not more, suffering for my animal friends as killing them for their flesh. I had become a vegetarian three years previously in mid-1994 when I made the conscious realisation between the life that once existed and the lamb's leg I was about to eat. I had no idea about the abhorrent treatments of chickens to get their eggs and cows to get their milk. Once I was aware of it I became vegan, as I didn't want to participate in the cruelty, abuse or death of any of the beings on this earth.

Vegans aim to do their part to end the suffering, cruelty and exploitation of all forms of animals by choosing not to use animals, their products or by-products for food, clothing and other purposes.

The word vegan was invented by Donald Watson in the 1940s but the term hadn't been widely used in the mainstream until the last decade. Vegans are committed vegetarians who choose to not eat animal flesh of any kind (including chickens and sea creatures), animal products (including eggs, dairy and honey) and by-products (including gelatine) as well as not wearing animal skins (leather) and animal products (silk, wool etc). Being vegan also means choosing compassionately with not only your food choices, but also fashion, cosmetics, household items; and not participating in events where animals will suffer or be exploited eg zoos and circuses.

Veganism is not a diet or a religion. Veganism is not about rules and regulations. It's not about constraints and fanaticism. It's about doing your part the best way you can to cause the least amount of suffering in this world. My main reason for adopting the vegan way of life is that I believe we should not use, kill or cause suffering to any (non-human) animals – especially when there are alternatives available. I believe in using our resources, whether it be material or mental, to create a positive environment for all of the creatures on earth. We are not like the non-human animals who kill in order to survive, as we have the ability to reason and act from a conscious level.

The main reasons most people become vegan are:

- Animal rights and welfare concerns
- Environmental and sustainable living
- Ethical and moral reasons
- Health issues
- Spiritual and/or religious beliefs
- Weight loss or control

I believe in speaking up whenever I see or hear of any injustices as well as not supporting companies that profit from exploitation. From social justice and human rights; to third world and poverty issues; to racial slurs and "jokes"; to feminist and gender equality issues; to fair trade and labour; to useable land and clean water for all of the earth; to overconsumption and waste; to anti-corporations and anti-multinationals. All of these are as important to me as anti-speciesism. Veganism is the best way for me to live a compassionate lifestyle in line with all of my ethics of anti-exploitation.

I am a committed vegan because I believe that we all need to tread as lightly as we can on the earth and to cause the least amount of pain and suffering to others while we're here. Veganism is the best thing that I can do and the best way I know how to lead by example to promote love, peace and compassion; and to stand against ALL injustices and exploitation that exist.

THE ENVIRONMENTAL CONSEQUENCES OF OUR DIETS

We don't all have to buy hybrid cars to help the environment when the adoption of a vegan diet is so much easier and cheaper. Doing both is even better.

Converting plant nutrients - including protein - to animal nutrients requires massive inputs of energy and water, and produces enormous amounts of greenhouse gases, including methane, which forms in the digestive system of ruminant animals such as cows, sheep and goats.

Depending on which factors are accounted for, estimates of livestock's share of greenhouse gas emissions range from just under 20% to around 50%.

The link between animal food products and climate change involves many inter-related factors, such as:

- Livestock's inherent inefficiency as a food source
- The massive scale of the industry, including tens of billions of animals slaughtered annually
- Land clearing and degradation
- Greenhouse gases, including carbon dioxide, methane and nitrous oxide
- Other warming agents, such as black carbon

Many official measures of greenhouse gas emissions under-report livestock's impact. The under-reporting has occurred because: relevant factors are omitted entirely from official figures (e.g. tropospheric ozone and black carbon); classified under different headings

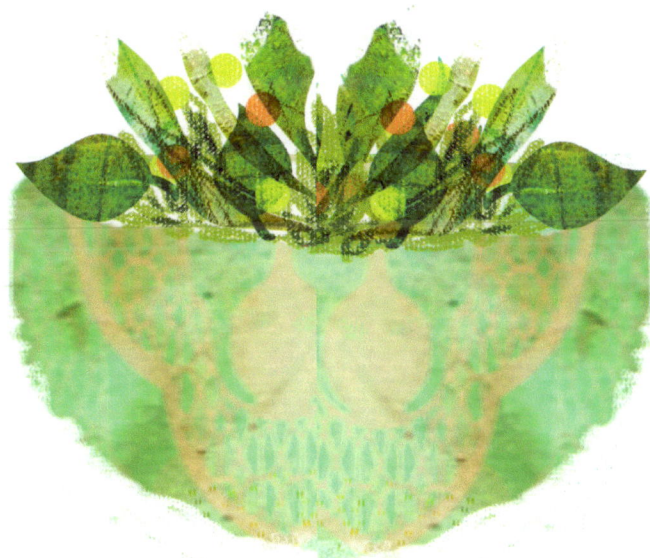

(e.g. livestock-related land clearing reported under "land use, land use change and forestry"); or considered but with conservative calculations (e.g. methane's impact based on a 100-year, rather than 20-year, "global warming potential").

(Source: 'Protecting Global Climate with Vegan Challenge' & 'Omissions of Emissions: A Critical Climate Change Issue' both by Paul Mahony)

THE BENEFITS OF VEGANISM

There are so many benefits to being vegan. To be able to look each non-human animal in the eye and know that they trust me is a very powerful and humbling experience. The advantage of feeling, being and actually looking healthy cannot be expressed fully in words. To know that you are doing your best to not contribute to any suffering of any other kindred spirit on this earth is a wonderful thought - plus you feel connected to all beings.

There are so many alternatives now to animal products that I find it laughable when people say that it's too hard to become vegan. Humans are very adaptable creatures and we change to fit our environment. When I first became vegan early in 1997 it was quite difficult to find vegan products and it was hard for me to give up mainstream chocolate and ice cream, but my reasons for doing so surpassed my cravings. There are so many supermarkets, locally owned stores as well as health food stores, markets and the vast amount of

The word vegetarian comes from the Latin word vegetare, which means - "to enliven."

vegan restaurants, websites and storefronts available now. There are many great quality alternatives to all animal products available, just do your research.

If you are not educated, become educated. Speak your truths whenever someone is listening. Encourage others to find their own truths and think outside of the mainstream boxes.

VEGAN HEALTH

The Academy of Nutrition and Dietetics says that, "[A]ppropriately planned vegetarian diets, including total vegetarian or vegan diets, are healthful, nutritionally adequate, and may provide health benefits in the prevention and treatment of certain diseases." To properly plan your diet, follow the basic guidelines below.

Vitamin B12 is the only nutrient not found in plant foods, so you should make sure you eat fortified foods or take a supplement on a regular basis. Once you have been vegan for awhile, you should take some time to

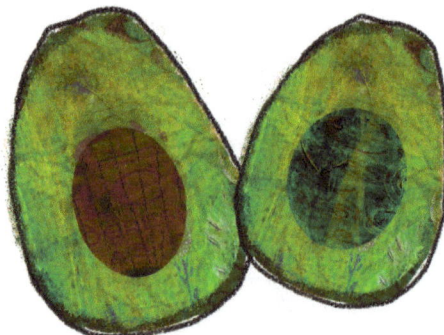

look into making sure all your nutrient needs are being met for the long term.

Be sure to consume the following every day:

- 5 or more servings of Grains and Starchy Vegetables
- 3 or more servings of Legumes, Soyfoods
- 1-2 servings of Nuts and Seeds
- 4 or more servings of Vegetables
- 2 or more servings of Fruits

(Source: 'Vegan for Life' book by Jack Norris, RD and Virginia Messina, MPH, RD)

FIRST, DO NO HARM

If you are compassionate, be compassionate. If not, then learn. Healing of the self comes from healing others and vice versa. If you do not contribute to any suffering towards any being on this earth, then you are contributing to the healing of the universe. Change your belief systems to change the world. Respect yourself and each other. Lead by example. Let your passions inspire all who come into your contact.

Surround yourself with positive people who are on the same life path as you, who dare to dream and aim to achieve. Do not waste your time and energies on negative people or people who thrive on creating or escalating drama. Don't force people who are not ready to change - their time will come - you cannot make them change. Small steps still get to the same destination. Take responsibility for all your actions and live your truths.

This is all for the voiceless.

Love and hugs,
Leigh-Chantelle xx

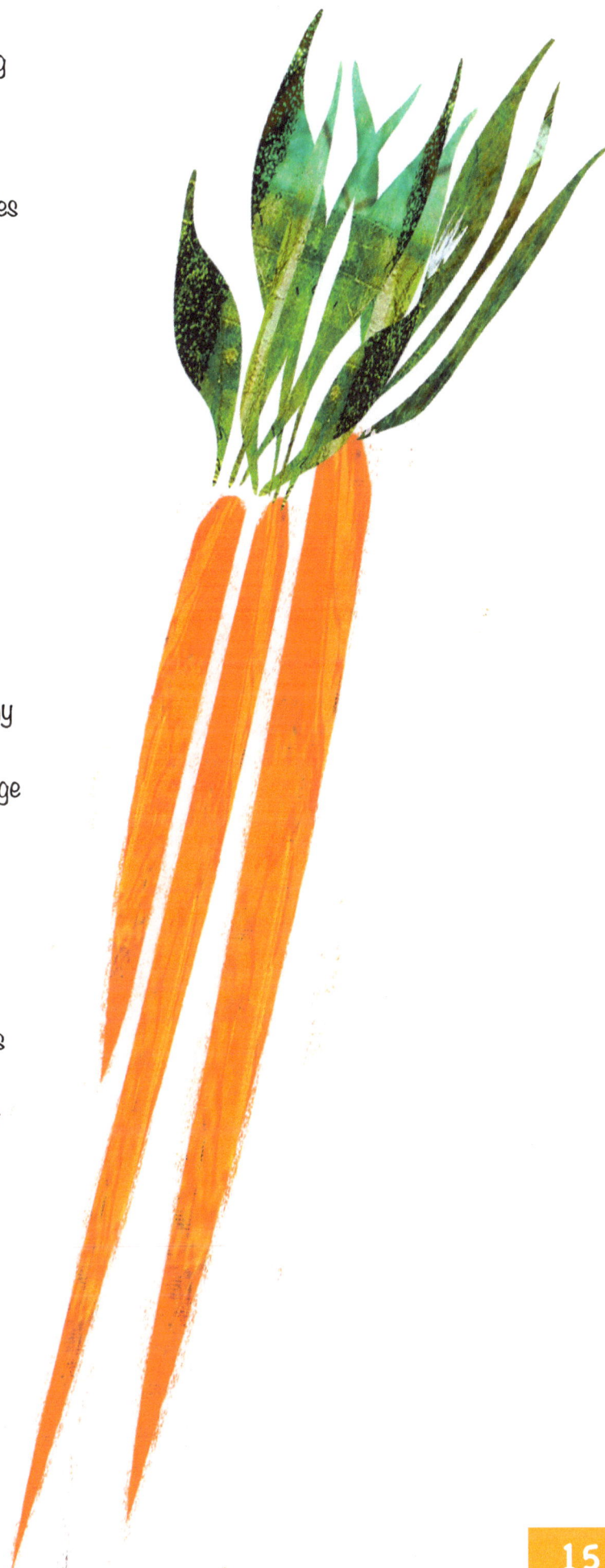

ingredients/Pantry List

FRUITS & VEGETABLES

Asparagus
Avocado
Beans (green)
Bean shoots
Broccoli
Brussels sprouts
Cabbage – red/purple and green
Capsicum (peppers) - red and green
Carrot
Celery
Chinese greens eg Bok choy,
    Chinese broccoli, Kai-lan, Pak choy
Corn
Currants
Dates
Eggplant (aubergine)
Figs
Garlic cloves
Lemon – juice, rind and flesh
Mushrooms – field
Nectarines

Okra
Olives – kalamata
Onion
Potato
Pumpkin
Snow peas (sugar snaps)
Spinach (silverbeet) & baby spinach leaves
Squash (marrows)
Sun-dried tomatoes
Sweet Potato (Kumara, similar to a Yam)
    – orange and purple
Tomatoes
Turnip (swede, rutabaga)
Zucchini (courgette)

GRAINS

Brown rice – medium and long grain
Couscous
Millet
Polenta (corn meal/semolina)
Quinoa – white and red
Rice flakes – thick (Indian)
Wild rice

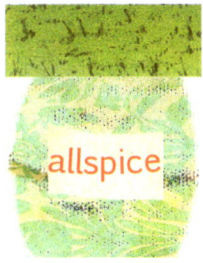

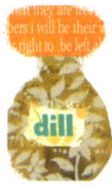

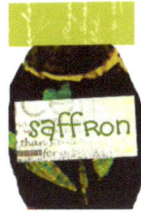

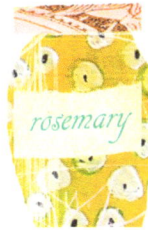

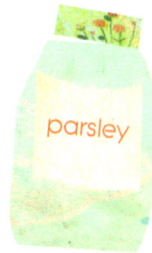

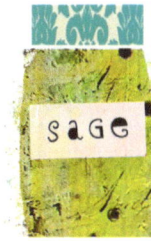

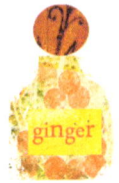

allspice

dill

saffron

rosemary

parsley

sage

ginger

HERBS

Basil
Cardamom
Cayenne pepper
Chilli
Coriander (cilantro)
Cumin
Dill
Ginger
Lemongrass
Oregano
Parsley
Peri Peri

NUTS & SEEDS

Almond, Brazil and Cashew spread
Almond – flakes and slivered
Cashews
Linseeds
LSA mix (linseed, sunflower and almond)
Peanut butter – crunchy
Pine nuts
Tahini (sesame seed paste) – unhulled
Walnuts

BEANS, LEGUMES & PULSES

Borlotti beans
Chickpeas (garbanzo beans)
Lentils
Red Kidney beans
Tempeh
Tofu – firm and silken (soft)

COLD ITEMS

Brown rice milk
Hummus
Soy cream cheese
Soymilk
Vegan/Soy margarine or butter

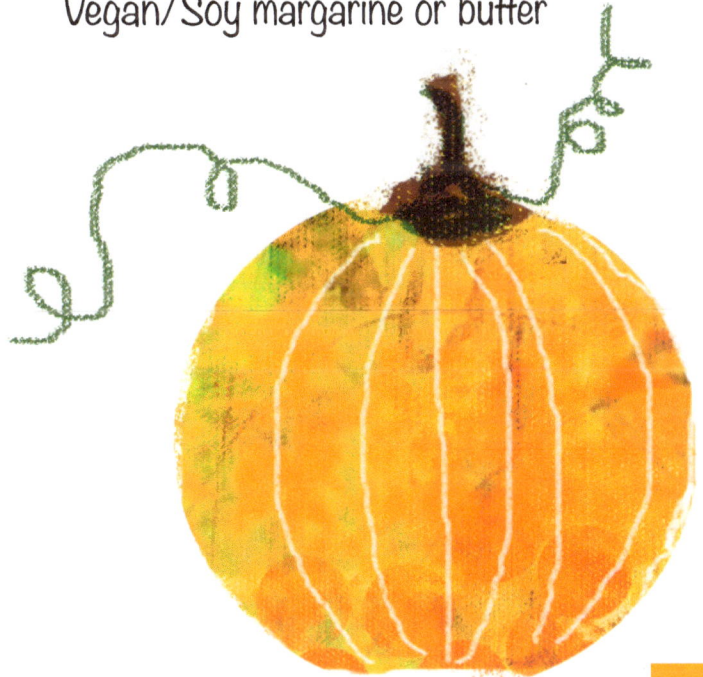

PANTRY ITEMS

Besan (chickpea) flour
Brown rice macaroni
Brown rice spirals
Buckwheat Pancake mix
Coconut Cream
Coconut - shredded
Extra Virgin Olive Oil
Falafels or Falafel mix
Filo pastry sheets
Flax Seed oil
Gnocchi
Hokkien noodles
Mung bean fettuccine
Pizza bases - gluten free
Rice and Corn Lasagne sheets
TVP (Textured Vegetable Protein)
 or vegan casserole mince

FLAVOURINGS

Cracked Black Pepper
Nutritional Yeast
Soy sauce or Tamari
Sweet chilli sauce
Vinegar

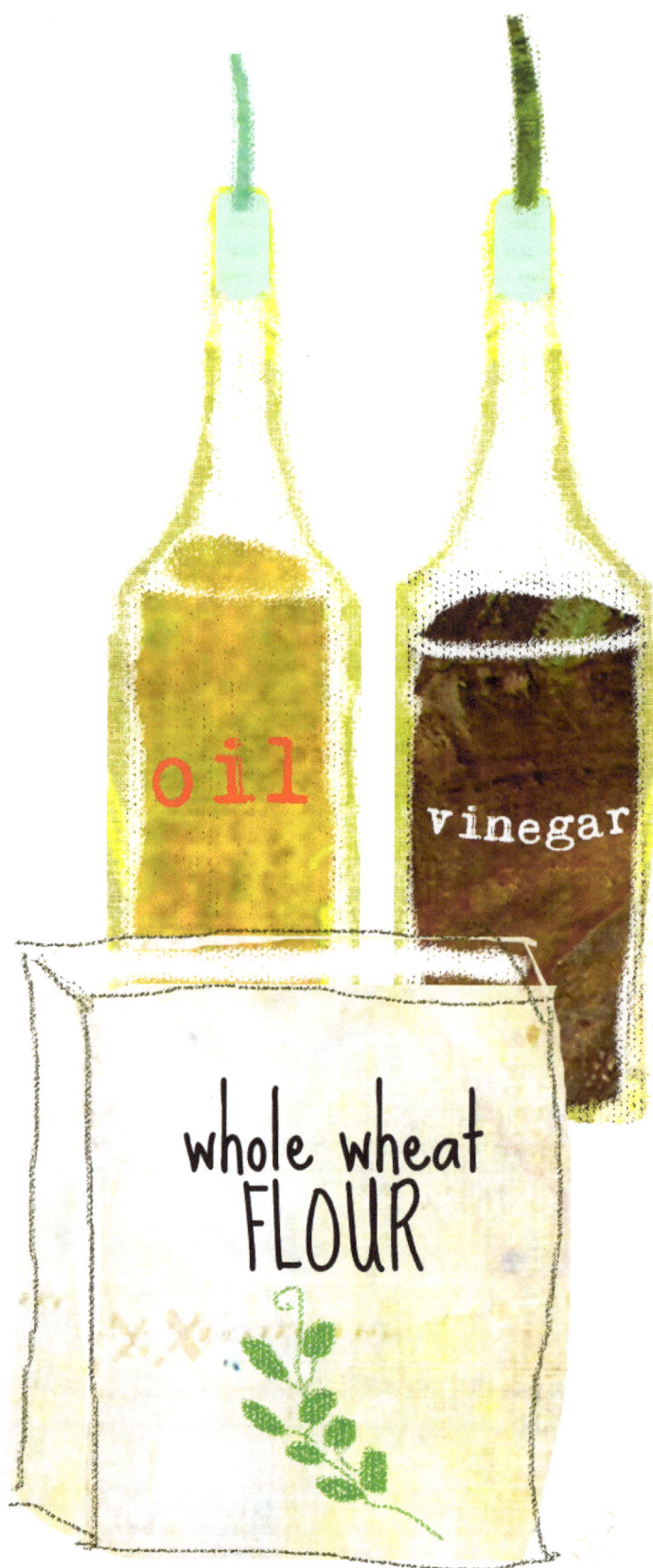

oil

vinegar

whole wheat
FLOUR

UTENSILS LIST

Baking dish - large
Bamboo Skewers
Casserole dish
Chopping board
Colander
Cooking/stirring utensils
Food processor (or a high-speed blender)
Fork
Frypan
Grill
Knives
Masher
Microwaveable bowl or jug
Mixing bowl
Oven/baking trays
Pastry brush
Pizza trays
Plastic bag – medium
Saucepan
Serving utensils
Sifter
Soufflé bowls or Ramekins
Spatula
Spoon
Steamer
Vegetable scrubbing brush
Whisk
Wok

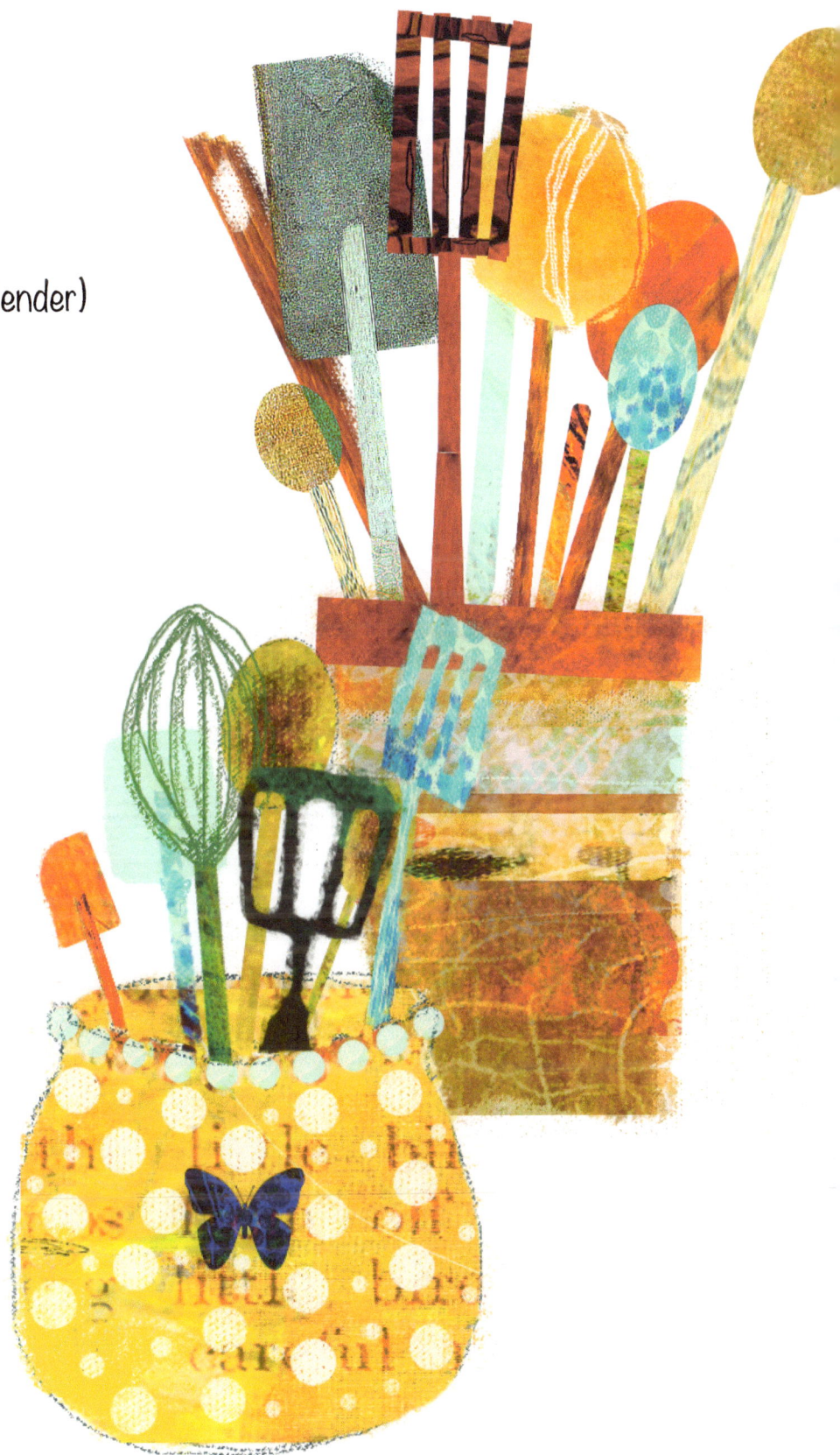

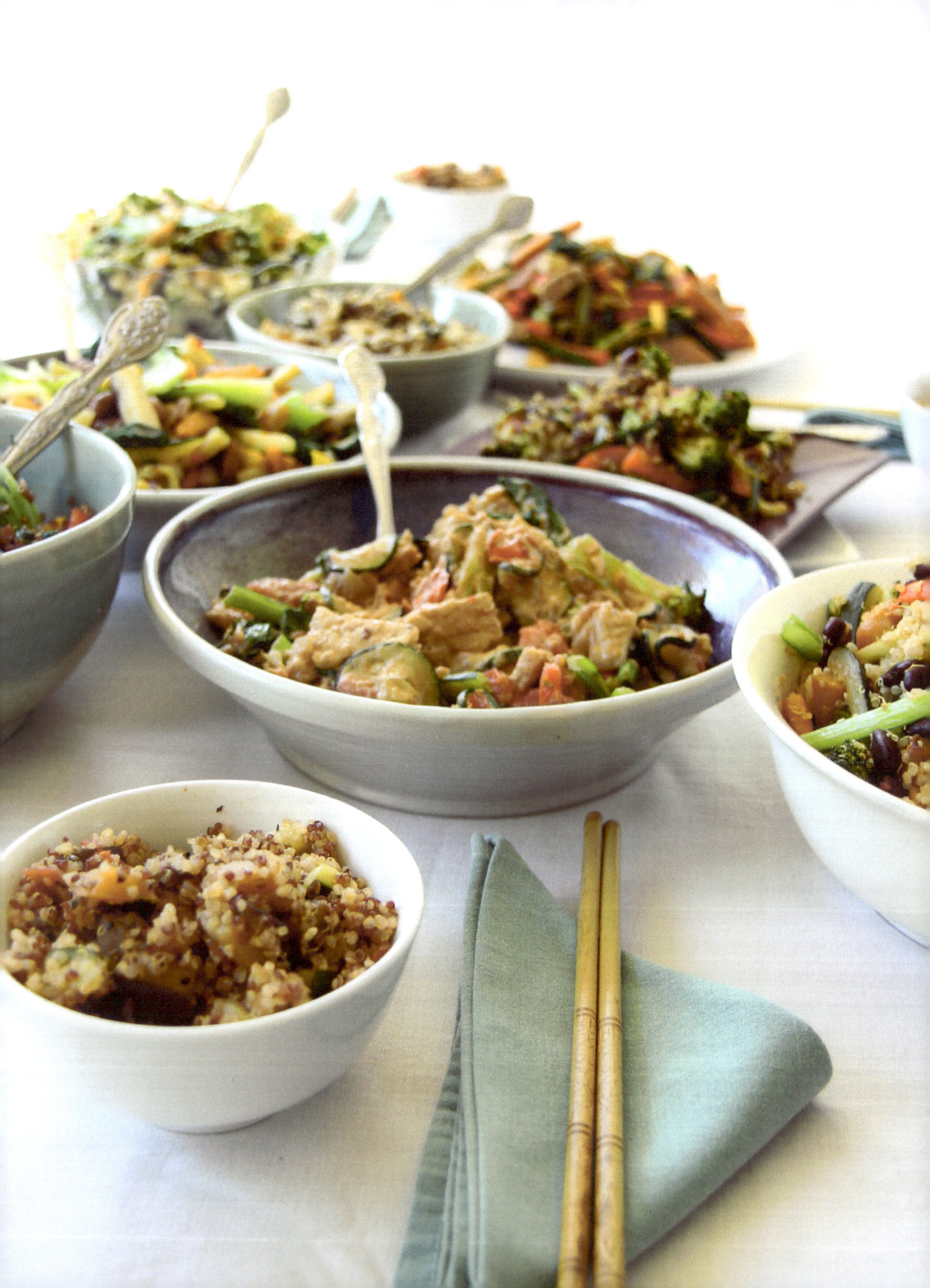

the Recipes

couscous and roasted vegetable salad

Serves 4-6 people NF

INGREDIENTS

½ red capsicum (pepper), cut in half
½ green capsicum (pepper), cut in half
½ eggplant (aubergine), sliced
½ sweet potato, sliced
6 field mushrooms, sliced
¼ pumpkin, sliced
2 zucchinis (courgette), sliced
2 cups couscous
¼ cup lemon juice and rind
1 ¾ cup water
1 tablespoon vegan margarine
1 garlic clove, crushed
2 tbsp vinegar
2 tbsp extra virgin olive oil
Handful of chopped parsley, basil and dill
Cracked black pepper

METHOD

- Brush all vegetables with extra virgin olive oil and grill each lot separately until cooked, remember to turn onto the other side
- Place grilled capsicum in a plastic bag to help remove the skin, leave for 5-10 minutes and peel off skins
- Let all vegetables cool, then dice the vegetables coarsely
- In a saucepan, boil water and lemon juice
- Remove from heat and stir in the couscous with a fork
- Cover the saucepan and allow to stand for 5 minutes while the couscous swells
- Place back on low heat and add margarine, stir for a few minutes with fork, separating the grains
- Combine the couscous with the chopped vegetables
- Mix together the oil, garlic, vinegar and pepper to season, add the chopped herbs and mix
- Add the liquid into the couscous and vegetables mixture and combine well.
- Serve chilled, with avocado as a salad, or as a filling in a roll, wrap or bread.

Live your beliefs and you can turn the world around.
- Henry Thoreau

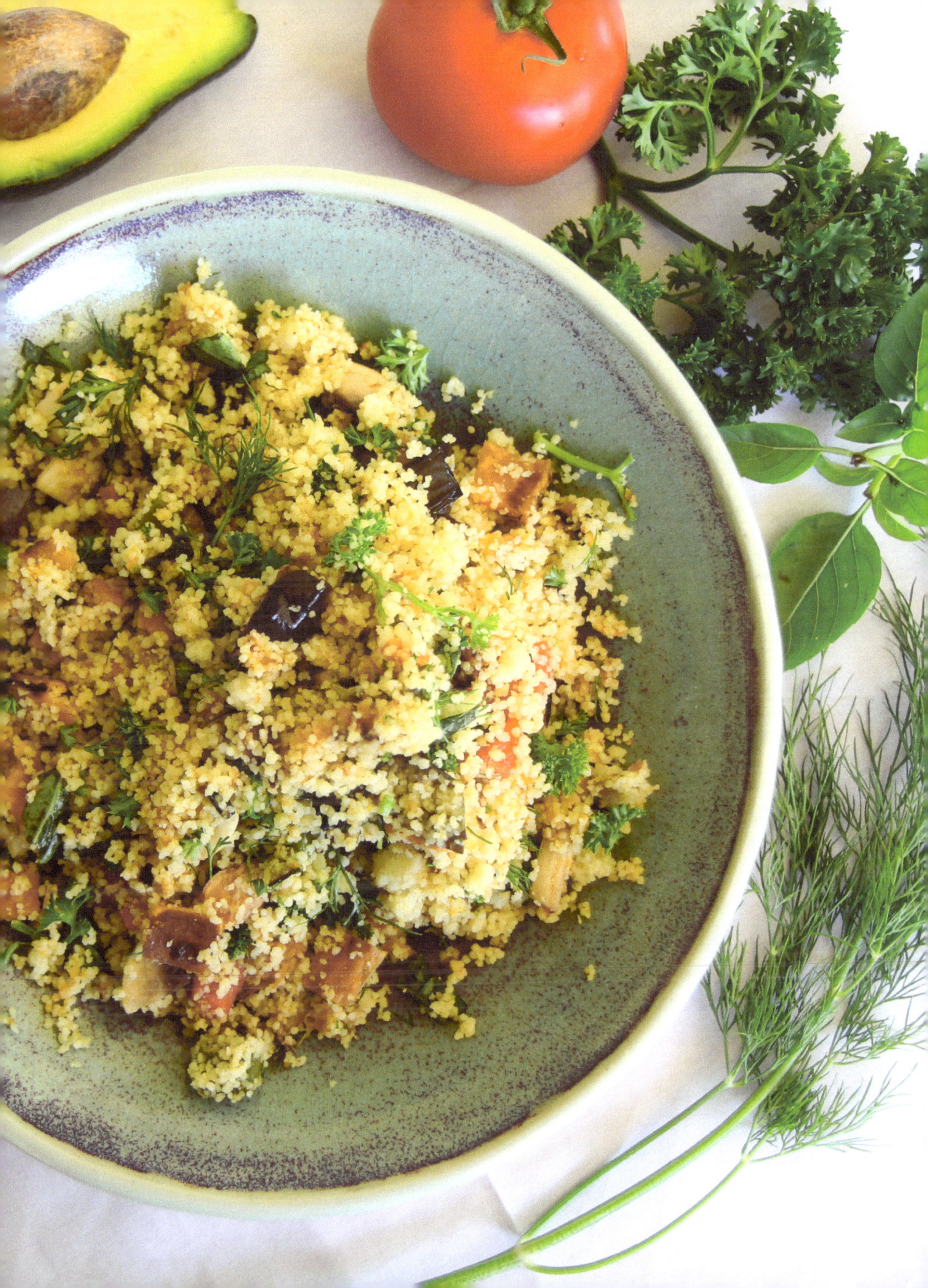

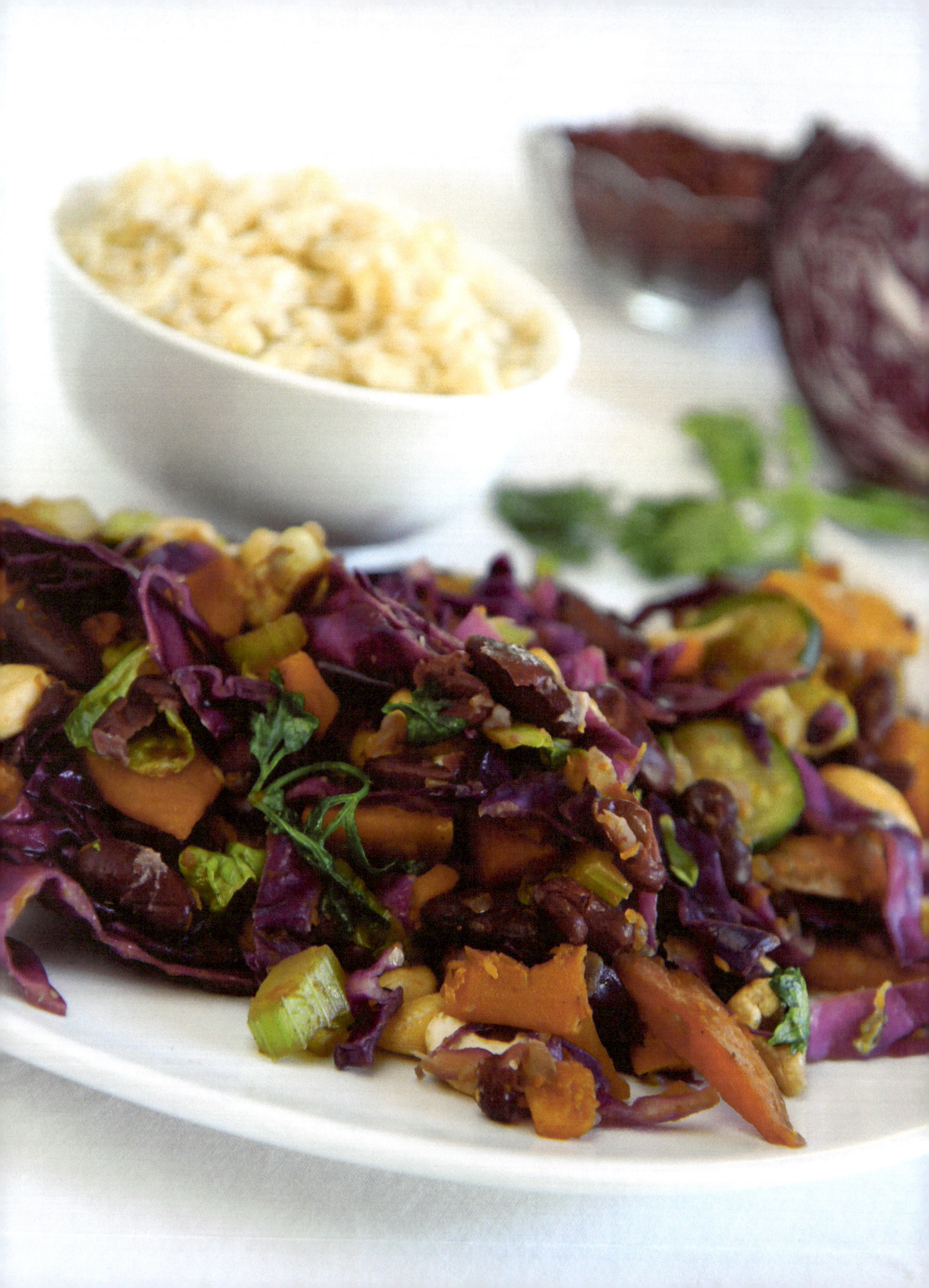

Stir-fry with red kidney beans

Serves 4 people GF SF

INGREDIENTS

1 celery stalk, chopped
½ sweet potato, cut into thin strips
8 Brussels sprouts, thinly sliced
¼ pumpkin, thinly sliced
1 zucchini (courgette), cut into thin strips
¼ red/purple cabbage, thinly sliced
2 garlic cloves, crushed
1 onion, thinly sliced
1 inch ginger, diced
400g red kidney beans, cooked
¼ cup cashews
Bunch of coriander (cilantro), chopped

METHOD

- Sauté garlic, onion and ginger in wok with oil
- Add celery, sweet potato, Brussels sprouts, pumpkin and zucchini
- Stir-fry until almost cooked
- Add cabbage, ensuring all ingredients are cooked
- Add cashews, coriander and red kidney beans
- Mix well and serve, with or without rice

Red kidney beans are great in soups, stir-fries, refried beans, in a chilli dish or salad. The red beans are a great addition to add colour to any recipe. Pulses need to be soaked overnight and then cooked or you can buy cans that are already cooked – just make sure that you rinse well before using.

Veganism may not be for the faint-hearted, for once we choose to respond in this way there's no turning back. It's as if we invest completely in conscience.
– David Horton

Mild curry with rice flakes

Serves 2-4 people GF SF

INGREDIENTS

1 cup thick (Indian) rice flakes
2 cups of filtered water
1 onion, diced
2 squash, diced
1 turnip, diced
1 sweet potato, diced
¼ pumpkin, diced
6 Brussels sprouts, diced
1 carrot, diced
400g lentils, cooked
200mL coconut cream
1 bunch of coriander (cilantro)
2 tbsp of lemongrass powder (or fresh)

METHOD

- Stir-fry all vegetables in a wok until semi-cooked
- Add lentils, herbs and coconut cream, mix thoroughly
- Bring to the boil and then simmer for 10-15 minutes
- Cook rice flakes in boiling water for 10-15 minutes
- Spoon cooked rice flakes into small soufflé bowls or ramekins and leave to set
- Place serving dish on top of soufflé bowls and tip over to serve
- Add vegetable and lentil mix onto the side of the rice flake cakes

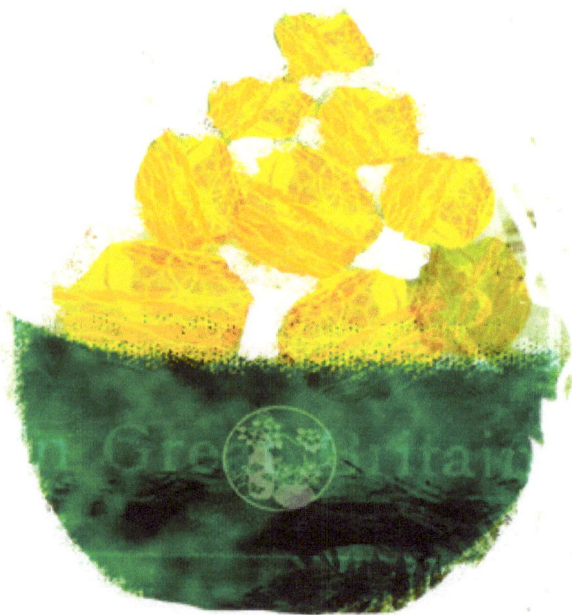

All wholesome food is caught without net or trap.
- William Blake

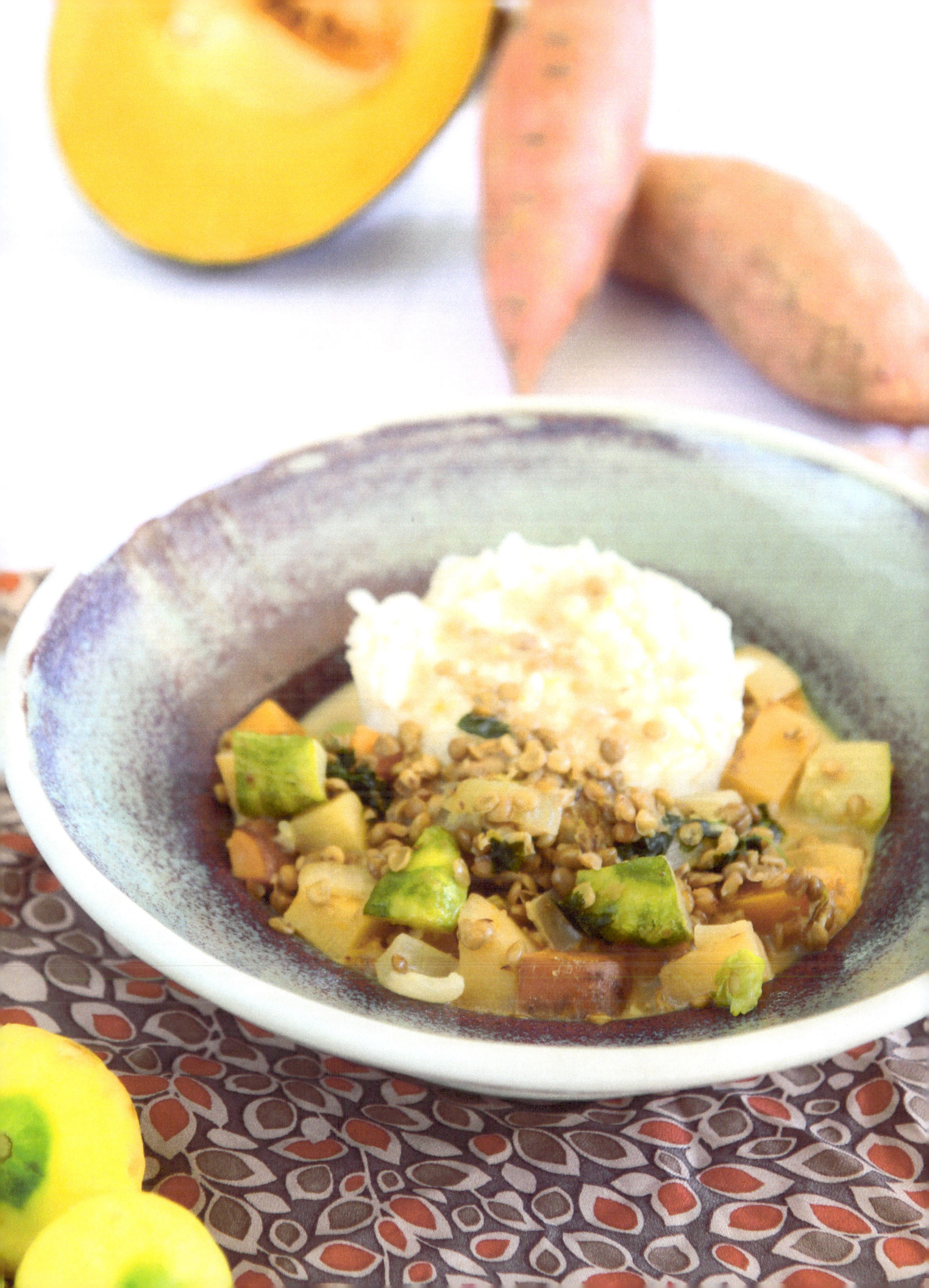

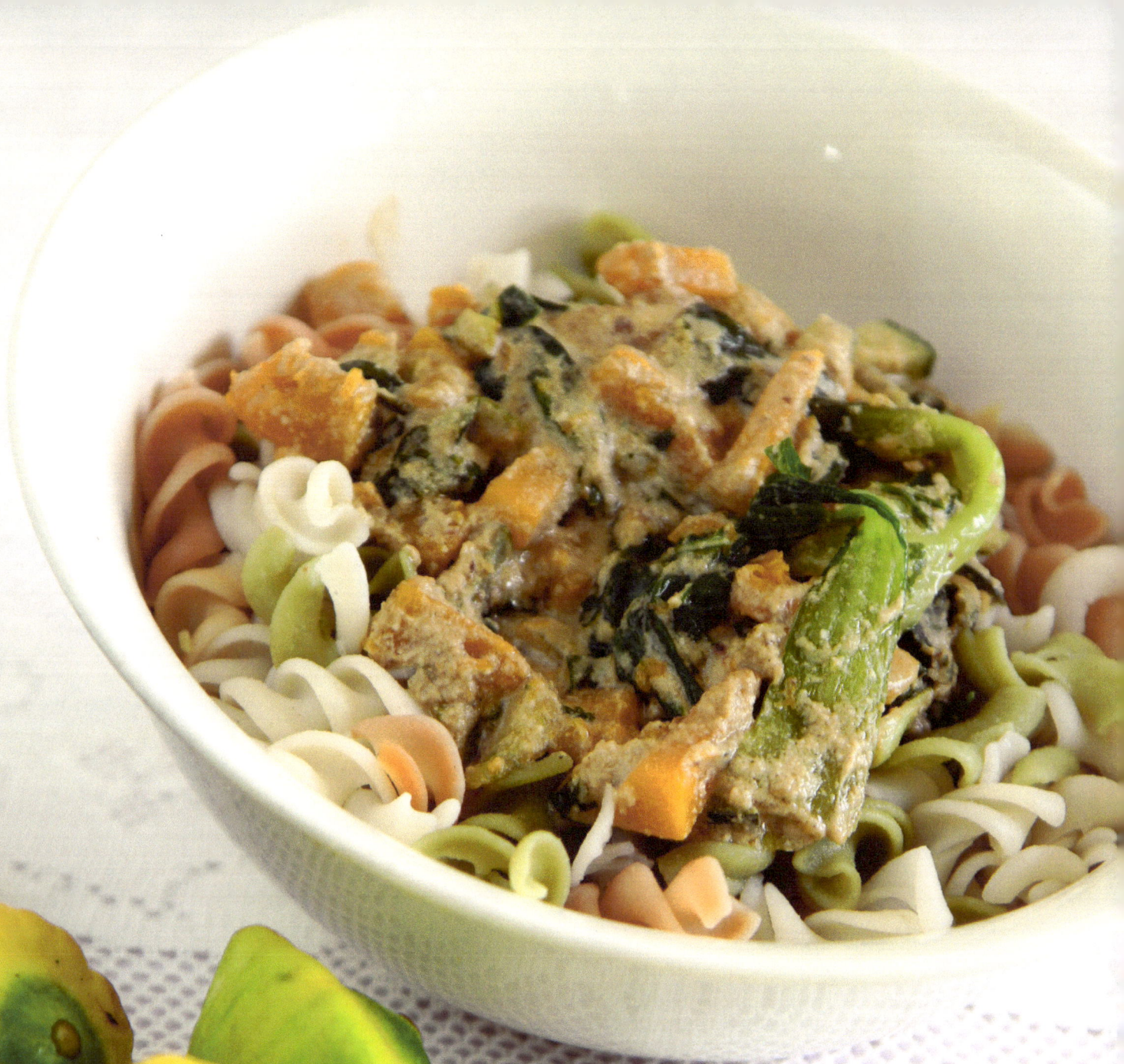

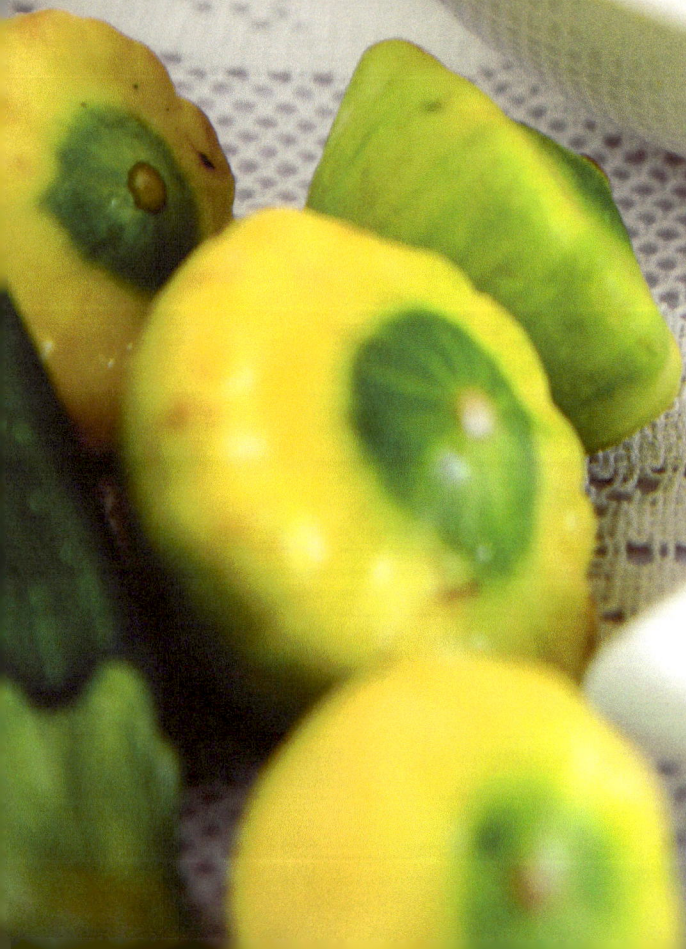

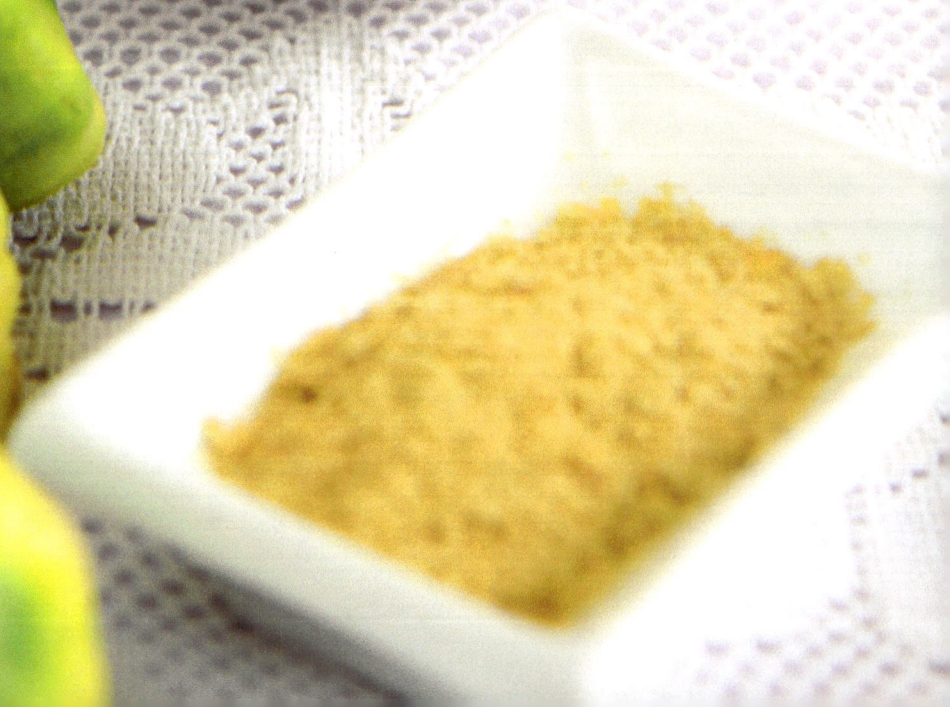

brown rice vegetable pasta

Serves 4-6 people `GF` `SF`

INGREDIENTS

250g Naked Foods Organic Brown Rice Spirals
2 zucchini (courgettes), thinly sliced
2 squash, thinly sliced
¼ pumpkin, thinly sliced
3 bunches of Chinese vegetables eg. bok choy, chopped
Coriander (cilantro) bunch, chopped
2 tbsp tahini
2 tbsp Melrose Almond, Brazil and Cashew spread
1 cup brown rice milk

METHOD

- Cook brown rice spirals in boiling water in a saucepan until soft
- Stir-fry zucchini, squash and pumpkin in wok until tender
- Combine tahini, nut spread and rice milk into paste in a separate container
- Add paste to wok and mix thoroughly
- Add Chinese vegetables and coriander, stir through until all cooked
- Combine with cooked pasta

Make your own spread by soaking ¼ cup each of almonds, Brazil nuts and cashews for a couple of hours. Combine in a food processor until smooth. Add a tablespoon of extra virgin olive oil or water if needed.

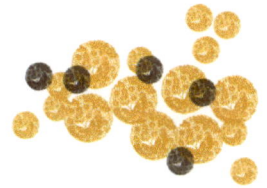

As long as there is conscious life on earth, there will be suffering. The question becomes what to do with the existence each of us is given. We can choose to add our own fury and misery to the rest or we can set an example by simultaneously working constructively to alleviate suffering while leading joyous, meaningful, fulfilled lives. Being a vegan isn't about deprivation or anger. It's about being fully aware so as to be fully alive.
- Matt Ball

sweet and sour quinoa

Serves 3-4 people `GF` `NF` `SF`

INGREDIENTS

1 cup of quinoa
2 cups of filtered water
1 zucchini (courgette), diced
6 tomatoes, diced
1 eggplant (aubergine), diced
6-8 nectarines, diced
4 tbsp oregano
2 tbsp cracked black pepper

METHOD

- Boil water in medium saucepan
- Add quinoa and cook until a white ring forms around the grain
- Cook tomatoes, oregano and black pepper in wok
- Add zucchini, eggplant and nectarines; stir-fry until cooked
- Stir through cooked quinoa and serve

Veganism isn't just a strict vegetarian diet; it is a complete philosophical viewpoint. It is practical in outlook, simple to understand and aspires to the highest environmental and spiritual values. I am sure it holds the key to a future lifestyle for a humane planetary guardianship.
- Howard Lyman

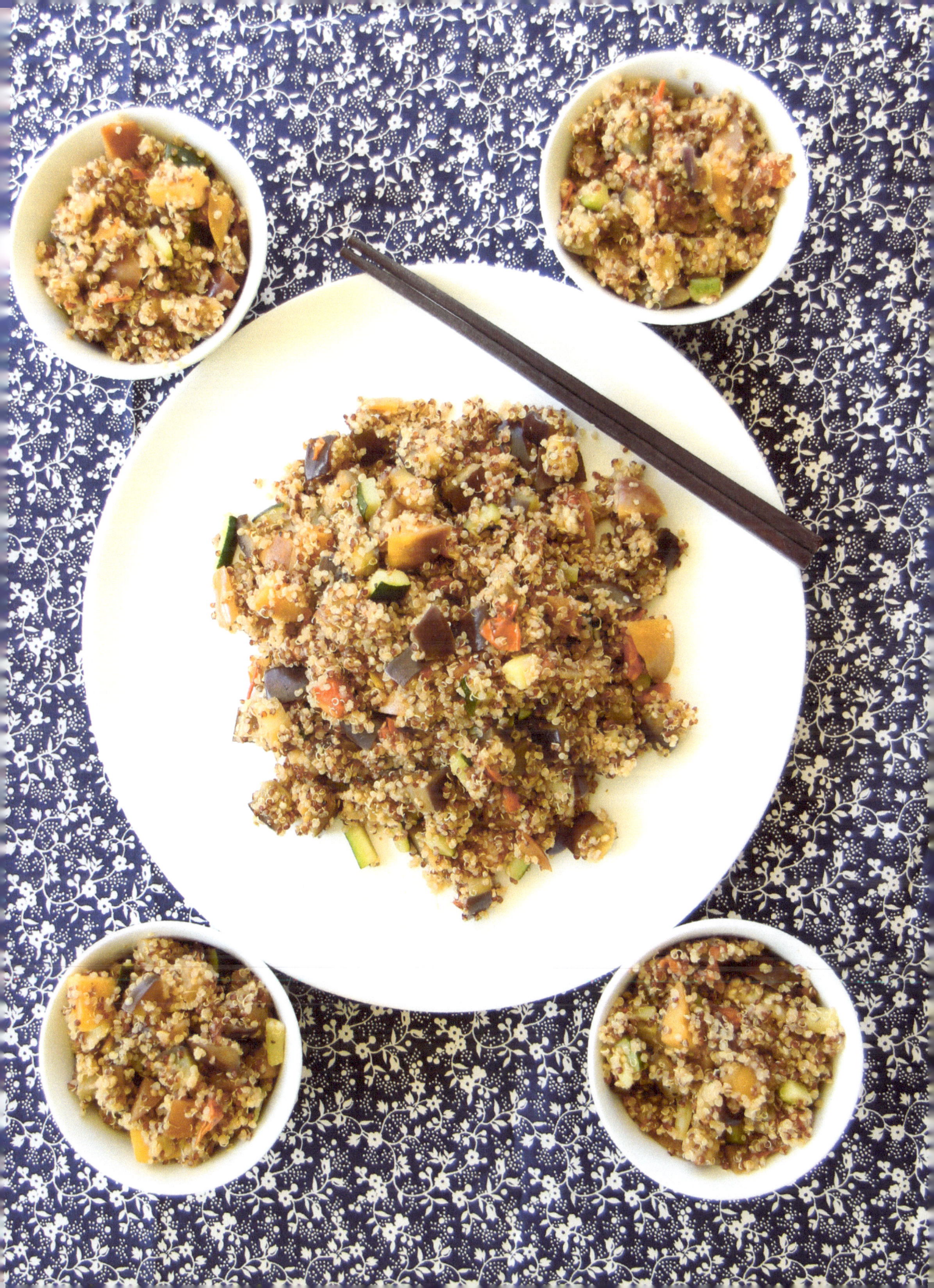

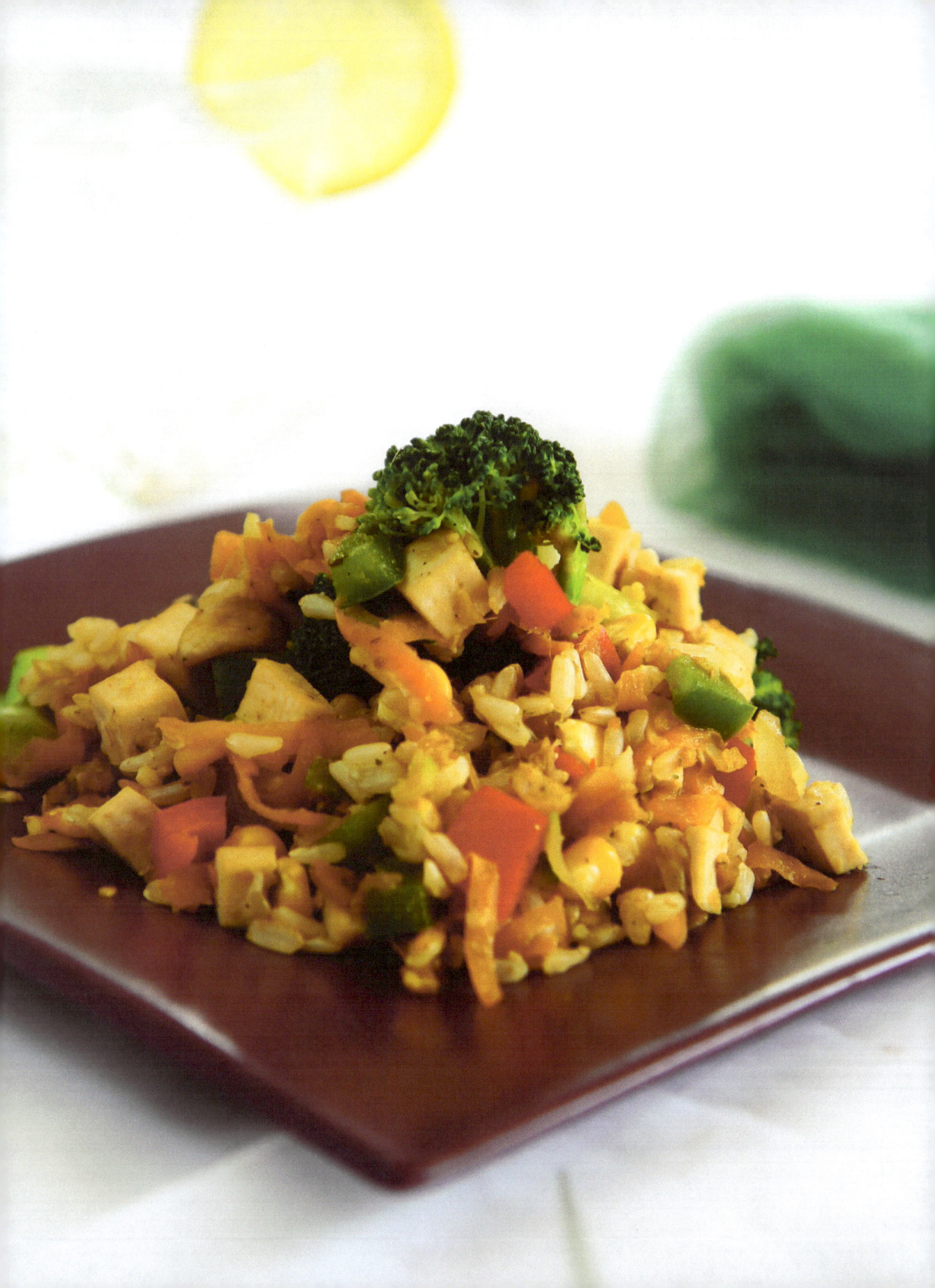

fried rice

Serves 4-6 people NF

INGREDIENTS

6 cups of filtered water
2 cups of brown rice
2 garlic cloves, crushed
1 onion, diced
Small amount of ginger, grated
1 cob of corn, kernels cut from the cob
1 zucchini (courgette), grated
1 carrot, grated
1 cup broccoli florets
½ red capsicum (pepper), diced
½ green capsicum (pepper), diced
¼ pumpkin, grated
8 mushrooms, diced
300g firm tofu, finely sliced
2 falafels, diced
Soy sauce or tamari

METHOD

- Cook brown rice in boiling water for about 30 minutes until tender
- Sauté garlic, onion and ginger in wok
- Add all vegetables into the wok and cook until tender
- Add tofu and falafel and mix well
- Combine cooked rice with the vegetable mixture
- Add soy sauce to taste
- Serve as a main meal or side dish
- Can be cooled and served as a salad

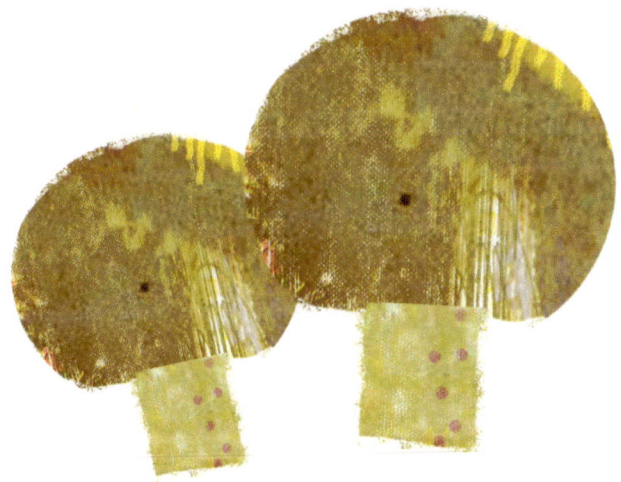

Until he extends the circle of his compassion to all living creatures, man will not himself find peace.
- Albert Schweitzer

curry puffs

Serves 4-6 people

INGREDIENTS

2 carrots, diced
1 eggplant (aubergine), diced
1 potato, diced
1 sweet potato, diced
6 field mushrooms, diced
1 red capsicum (pepper), diced
2 zucchinis (courgette), diced
¼ pumpkin, diced
415g (can) Sanitarium casserole mince or
    Textured Vegetable Protein (TVP)
200mL coconut cream
1 onion, diced
1 garlic clove, crushed
1 packet of Antoniou filo pastry
1 cup of shredded coconut
1 tsp coriander (cilantro)
1 tsp chilli
1 tsp cayenne pepper
1 tsp cardamom
1 tsp cumin
1 tsp peri peri
(Use only ½ tsp of each spice if you don't like too spicy!)
Sweet chilli sauce to serve
Extra virgin olive oil, heated when needed

METHOD

- Pre-heat oven to 210°C (410°F)
- Mix the spices, casserole mince and coconut cream together - set aside
- In a wok, sauté garlic and onion with a splash of oil
- Stir-fry vegetables until mostly cooked
- Add casserole mince and coconut cream mixture, simmer for 10 minutes
- Add coconut then allow mixture to cool down
- Brush one side of the filo pastry with oil and fold together, brush half and fold again
- On the diagonal filo sheet, spoon mixture onto the lower right hand corner and fold diagonally until the end, oil to seal – see the diagram
- Brush outside of curry puffs with oil
- Cook in a hot oven 210°C (410°F) until golden
- Serve with sweet chilli sauce

The animals of the world exist for their own reasons. They were not made for humans any more than black people were made for white, or women created for men.
- Alice Walker

how to fold:

1. fold in half

2. fold in half again

3. spoon on filling

fold diagonally brush with oil

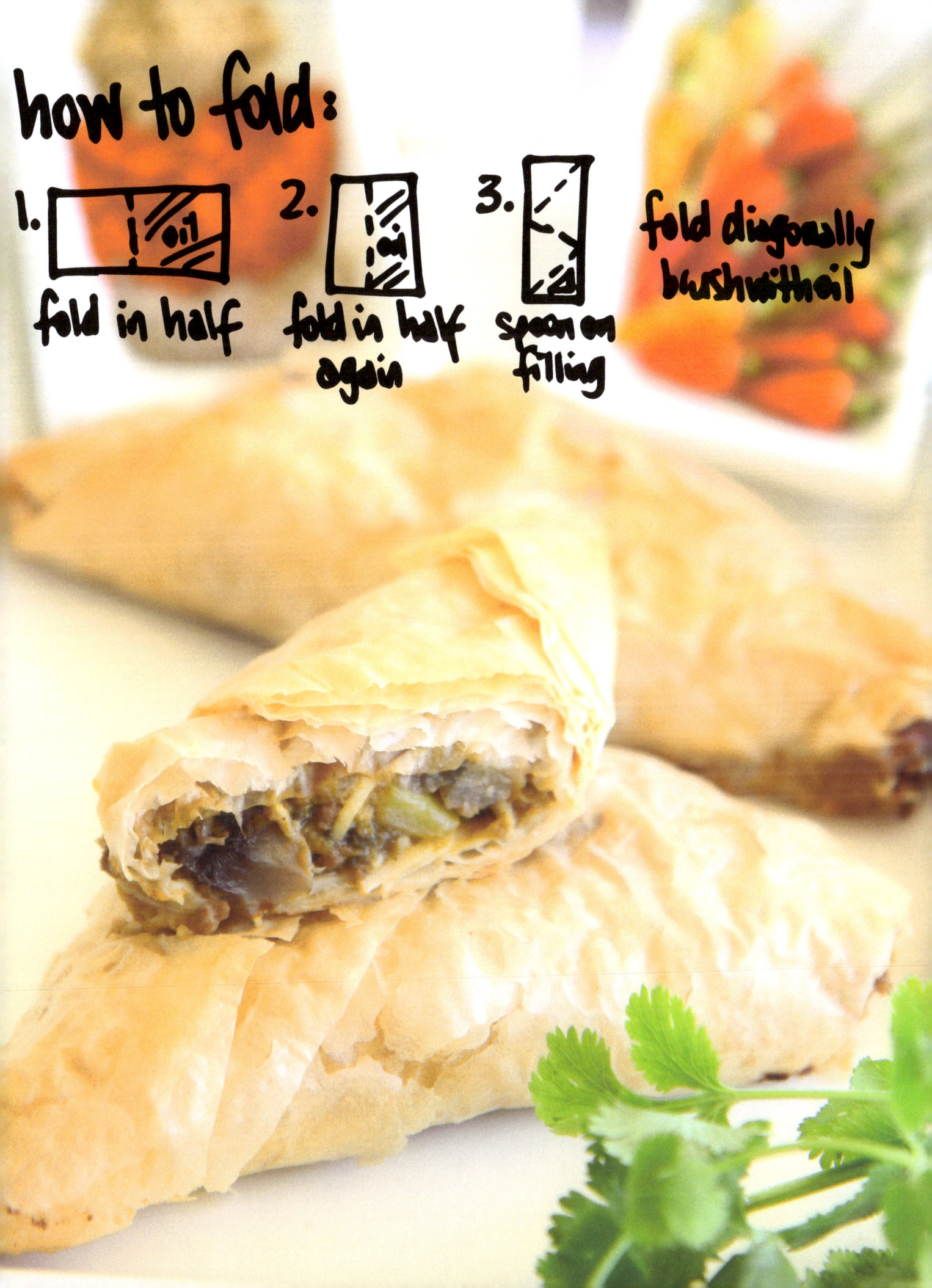

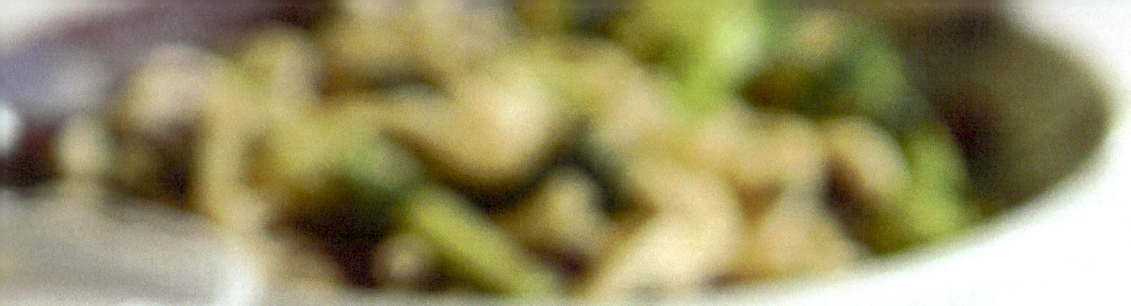

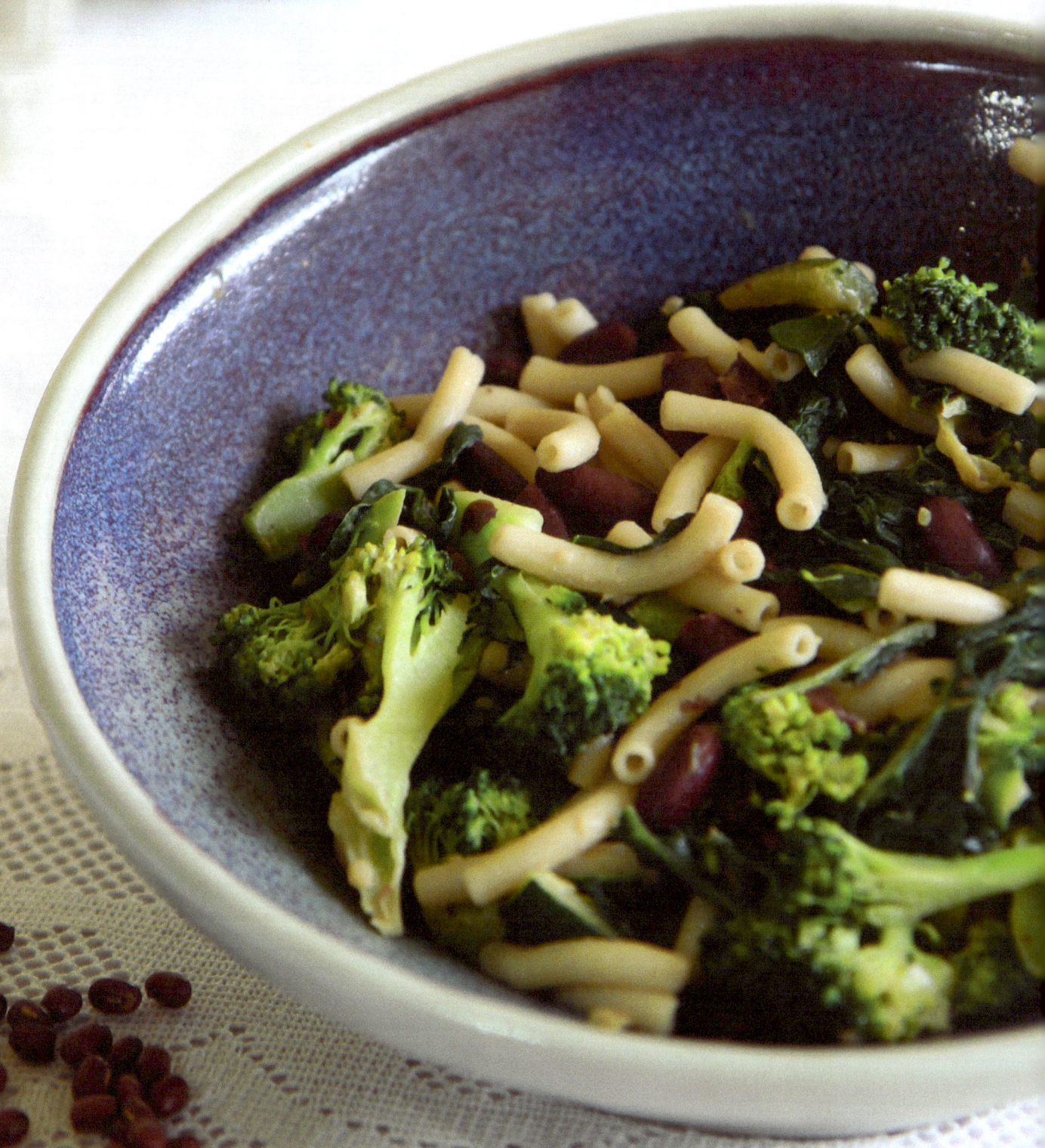

kidney bean macaroni

Serves 4-6 people GF NF

INGREDIENTS

350g Berconia brown rice macaroni
2 zucchinis (courgettes), cut into thin strips
2 cups of broccoli florets
½ bunch of spinach, coarsely chopped
400g red kidney beans, cooked
2 garlic cloves, crushed
Extra virgin olive oil
4 tbsp soy cream cheese

METHOD

- Bring a large saucepan of water to boil
- Add brown rice macaroni
- Boil until cooked, approx 10-15 minutes
- Sauté garlic and oil in wok
- Add zucchini, broccoli and spinach
- When cooked stir through red kidney beans and cooked macaroni
- Stir through soy cream cheese when still hot

In separateness lies the world's great misery; in compassion lies the world's true strength.
- Buddha

millet and tempeh stir-fry

Serves 3-4 people GF NF

INGREDIENTS

1 cup of millet
2 cups of filtered water
1 zucchinis (courgettes), thinly sliced
4 okras, sliced in quarters lengthwise
1 red capsicum (pepper), sliced lengthwise
4 large spinach leaves, coarsely chopped
200g tempeh, sliced
2 garlic cloves, crushed
Small amount of ginger, grated
Handful of coriander (cilantro), finely chopped
Extra virgin olive oil

METHOD

- Bring water to boil in a medium saucepan
- Cook millet until all water is absorbed, use fork to separate grains
- Sauté garlic and ginger with oil in wok
- Add zucchini, okra and capsicum; stir-fry until cooked
- Stir through spinach, coriander and tempeh
- Add cooked millet to the mix and serve

Millet is a great rice alternative, gluten-free and high in protein and magnesium. It has a similar consistency to couscous and can be used in porridges, soups, breads and stir-fries.

I expect to pass through this world but once; any good thing therefore that I can do, any kindness that I can show to any fellow creature, let me do it now; let me not defer to neglect it, for I shall not pass this way again.
- Etienne De Grellet

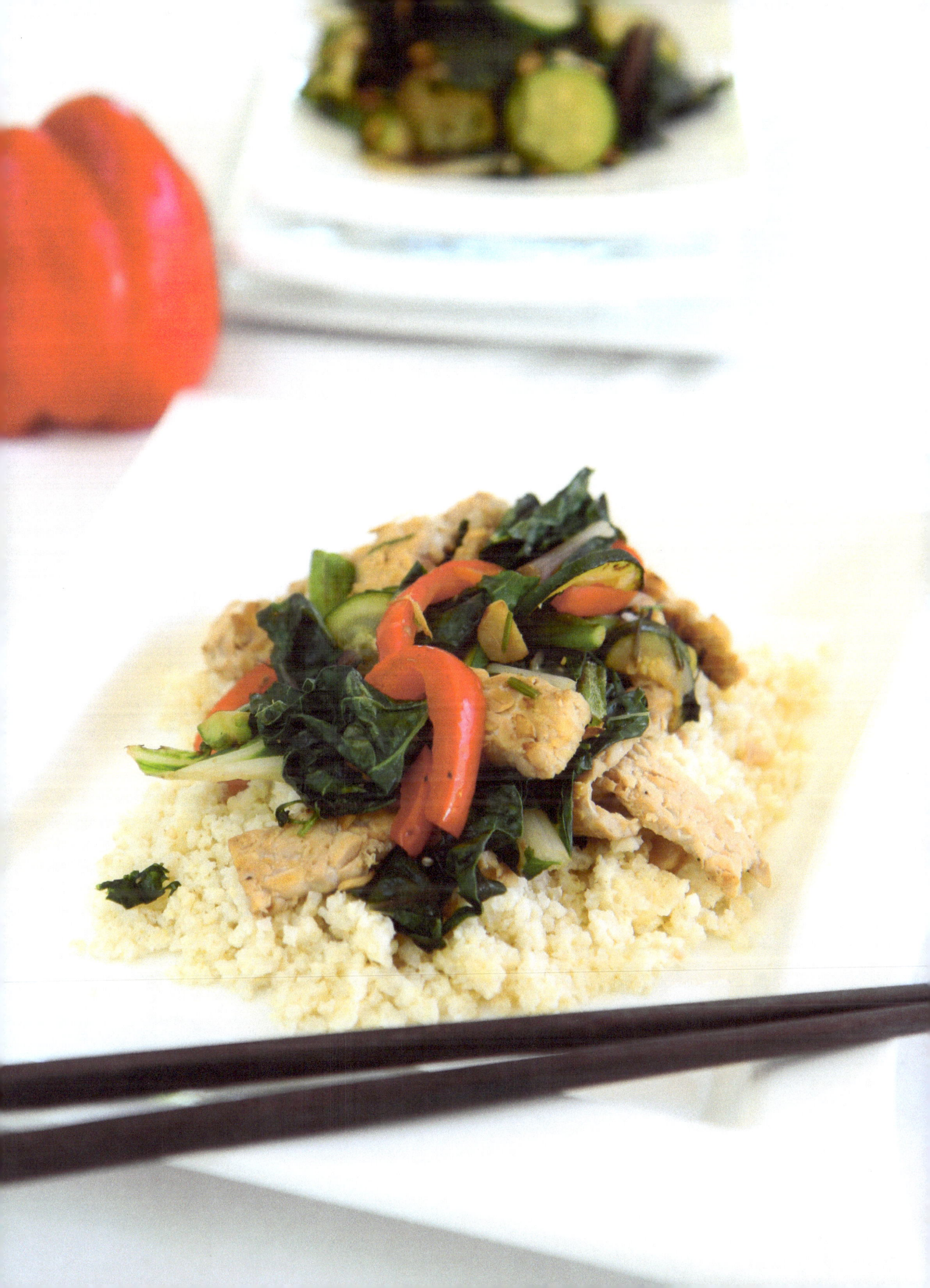

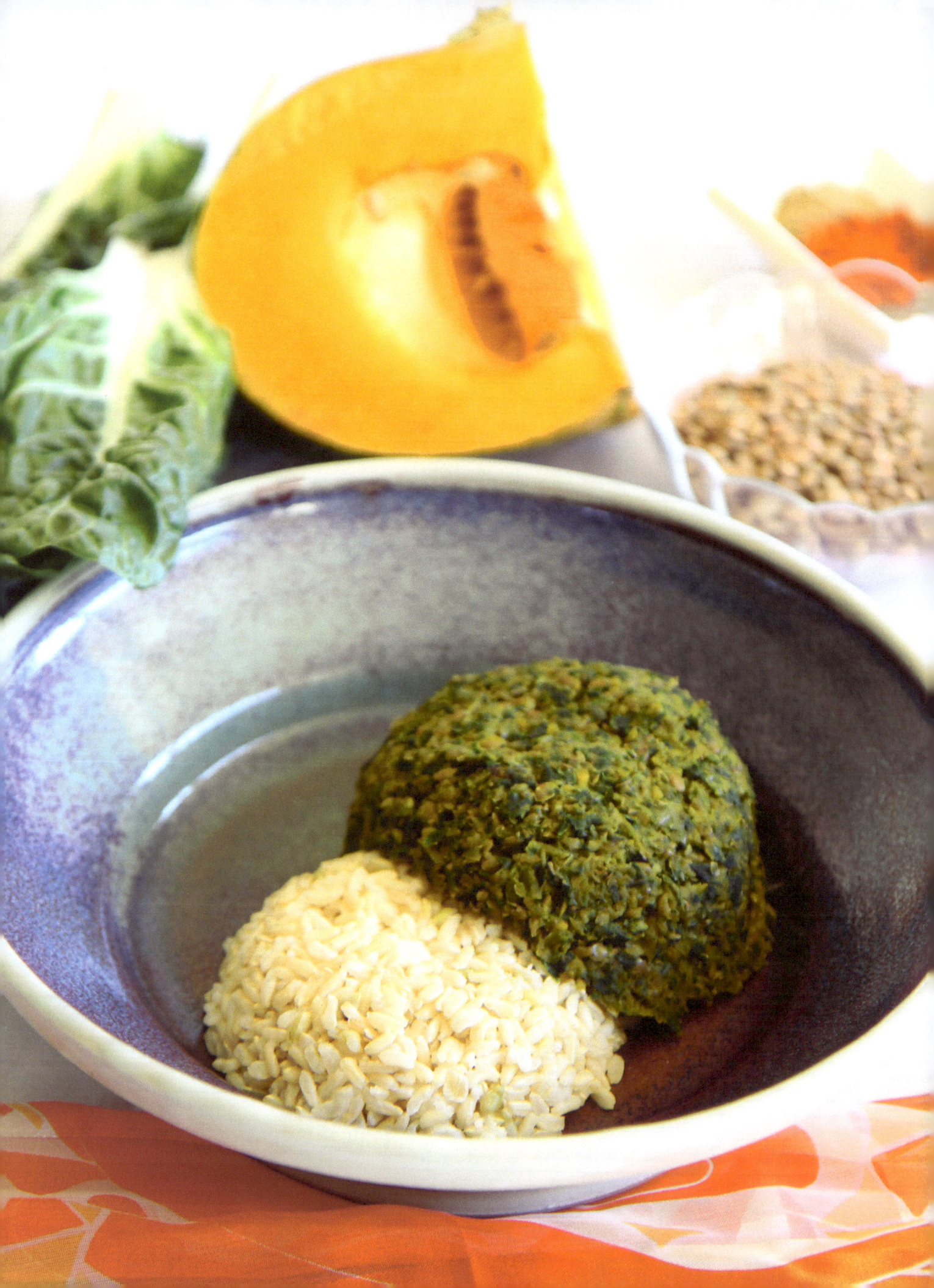

lentil and spinach curry

Serves 4-6 people GF NF SF

INGREDIENTS

1 onion
2 garlic cloves
1 tsp cayenne pepper
1 tsp peri peri powder
1 tsp cardamom seed powder
1 bunch of spinach, stalks removed
¼ pumpkin
400g lentils, cooked

METHOD

- In a food processor, process the onion, garlic and spices
- Add mixture to lightly oiled wok and sauté
- Process the spinach, pumpkin and lentils and add to the wok
- Stir-fry until cooked
- Serve with brown rice along with soy yoghurt or soy cream cheese

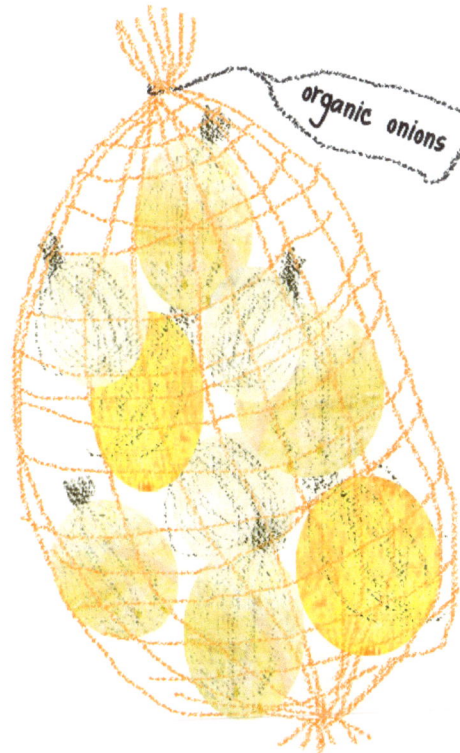

organic onions

Mercy begins with the smallest creature, and peace cannot exist without us until it exists within.
- Daharja

hokkien noodles

Serves 3-4 people **NF**

INGREDIENTS

2 cloves of garlic, crushed
1 onion, diced
1 cob of corn, kernels cut off
1 carrot, grated
1 pack of baby spinach leaves
½ red capsicum (pepper), diced
½ green capsicum (pepper), diced
375g pack of firm tofu, cut into thick slices
1 pack of hokkien noodles
Sweet chilli sauce
Extra virgin olive oil
¼ cup of LSA (Linseed, Sesame and Almond) mix

METHOD

- Sauté garlic and onion in wok with olive oil
- Add all vegetables except spinach and stir-fry until tender
- Add tofu and sweet chilli sauce
- Add spinach and separated hokkien noodles, gently cook until spinach is limp
- Take off the heat, add LSA mix, mix thoroughly and serve

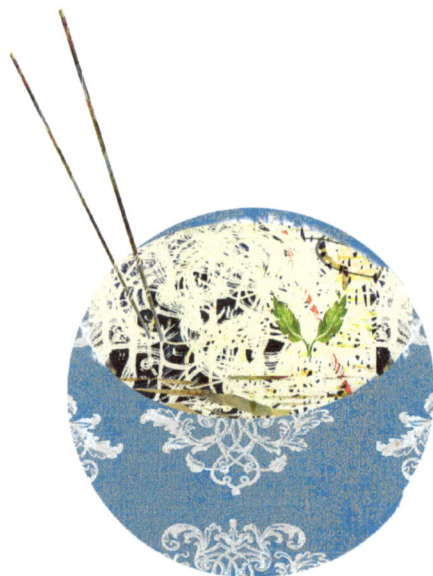

Sometimes the word evolution is used as a way to justify our actions.
- Stuart Andrews

42

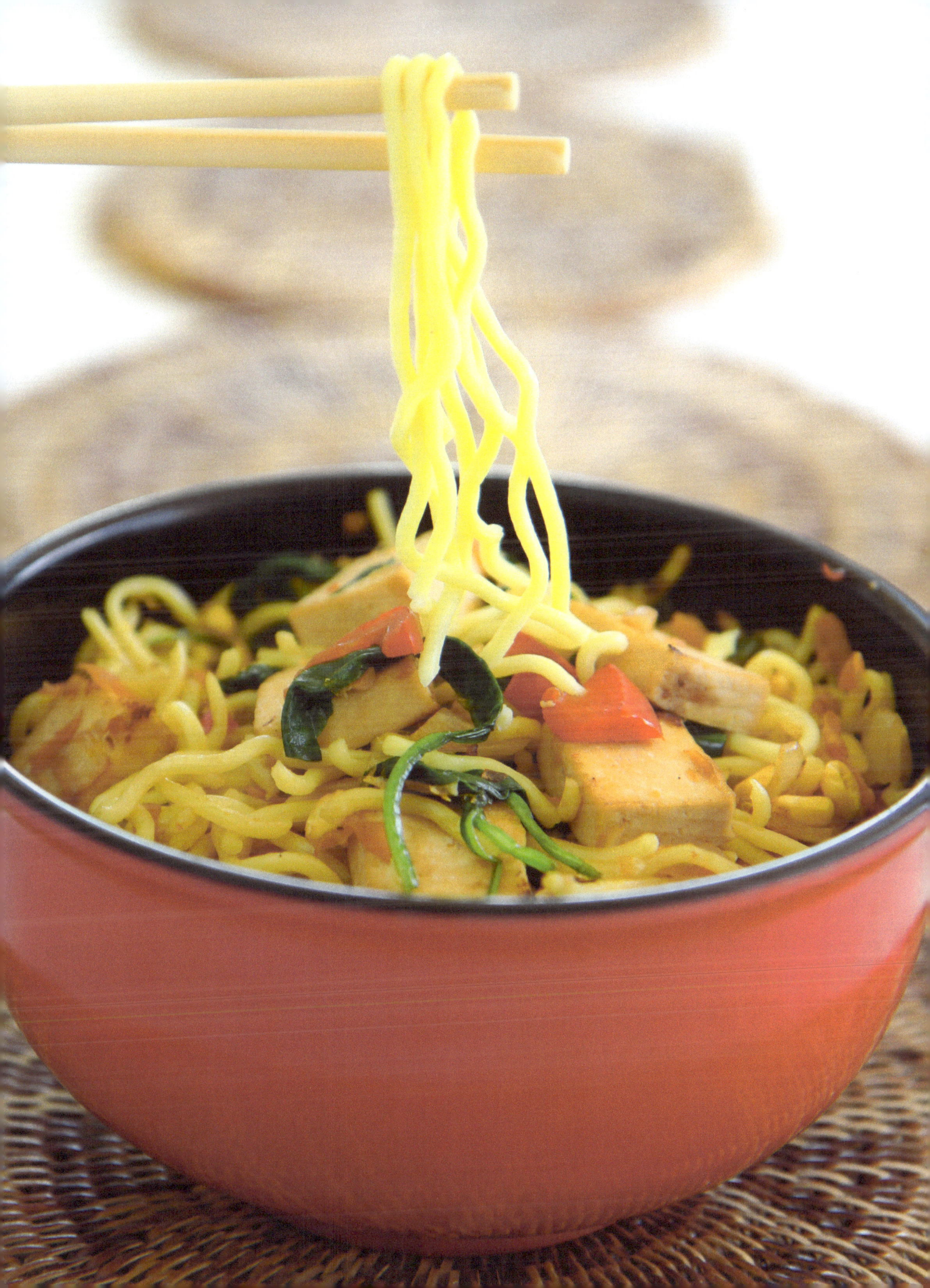

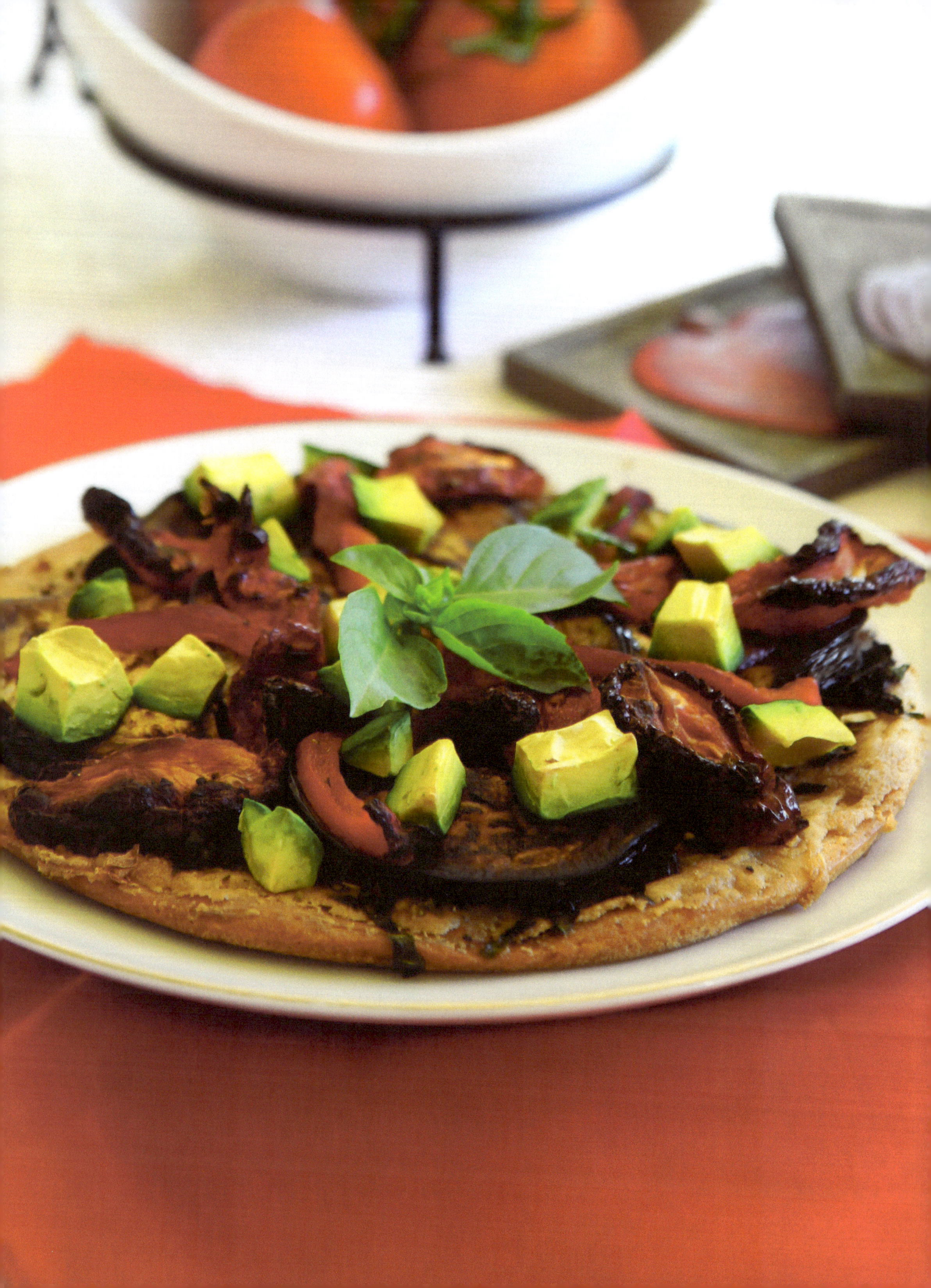

eggplant pizza

Serves 2 people GF NF

INGREDIENTS

1 large or 2 small gluten-free pizza bases
2 garlic cloves, crushed
Tahini
1 avocado
Soy cream cheese
Oregano
Basil
Cracked black pepper
¼ eggplant (aubergine), thinly sliced
¼ red capsicum (pepper), thinly sliced
50g semi-dried tomatoes

METHOD

- Thaw out pizza bases if necessary
- Spread tahini and soy cream cheese onto pizza bases
- Sprinkle garlic and spices over the bases
- Cut avocado in half, dice and leave to place on the pizza when almost cooked or spread one half onto each base
- Layer eggplant, capsicum and tomatoes onto bases
- Cook in medium oven 200°C (390°F) for 15-20 minutes
- Serve with warm rye garlic bread and salad

Life is life - whether in a cat, a dog, or man. There is no difference there between a cat or a man. The idea of difference is a human conception for man's own advantage.
- Sri Aurobindo

45

inca red quinoa stir-fry

Serves 3-4 people `GF` `NF` `SF`

INGREDIENTS

1 cup Inca red quinoa
2 cups filtered water
1 eggplant (aubergine), thinly sliced
4 yellow squash, thinly sliced
1 zucchini (courgette), thinly sliced
½ red capsicum (pepper), thinly sliced
1 bunch bok choy, coarsely chopped
2 garlic cloves, crushed

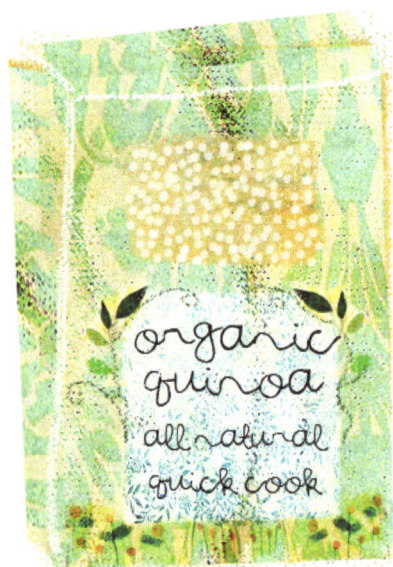

METHOD

- Cook quinoa and water in saucepan until white rims form on the periphery of the grain
- Sauté garlic cloves in a small amount of water
- Stir-fry eggplant, squash, zucchini and capsicum until tender
- Add bok choy, stir-fry until cooked
- Combine with quinoa and serve

Quinoa (pronounced Keen-wa) is an ancient seed (not really a grain) from the Inca civilisation. Quinoa is a complete protein and contains more protein than other grains. Quinoa is beautiful and comes in white, red and black. When it's cooked, a white rim forms on the periphery of the grain.

organic quinoa all natural quick cook

To be vegetarian is to disagree - to disagree with the course of things today. Starvation, world hunger, cruelty, waste, wars - we must make a statement against these things. Vegetarianism is my statement. And I think it's a strong one.
- Isaac Bachevis Singer

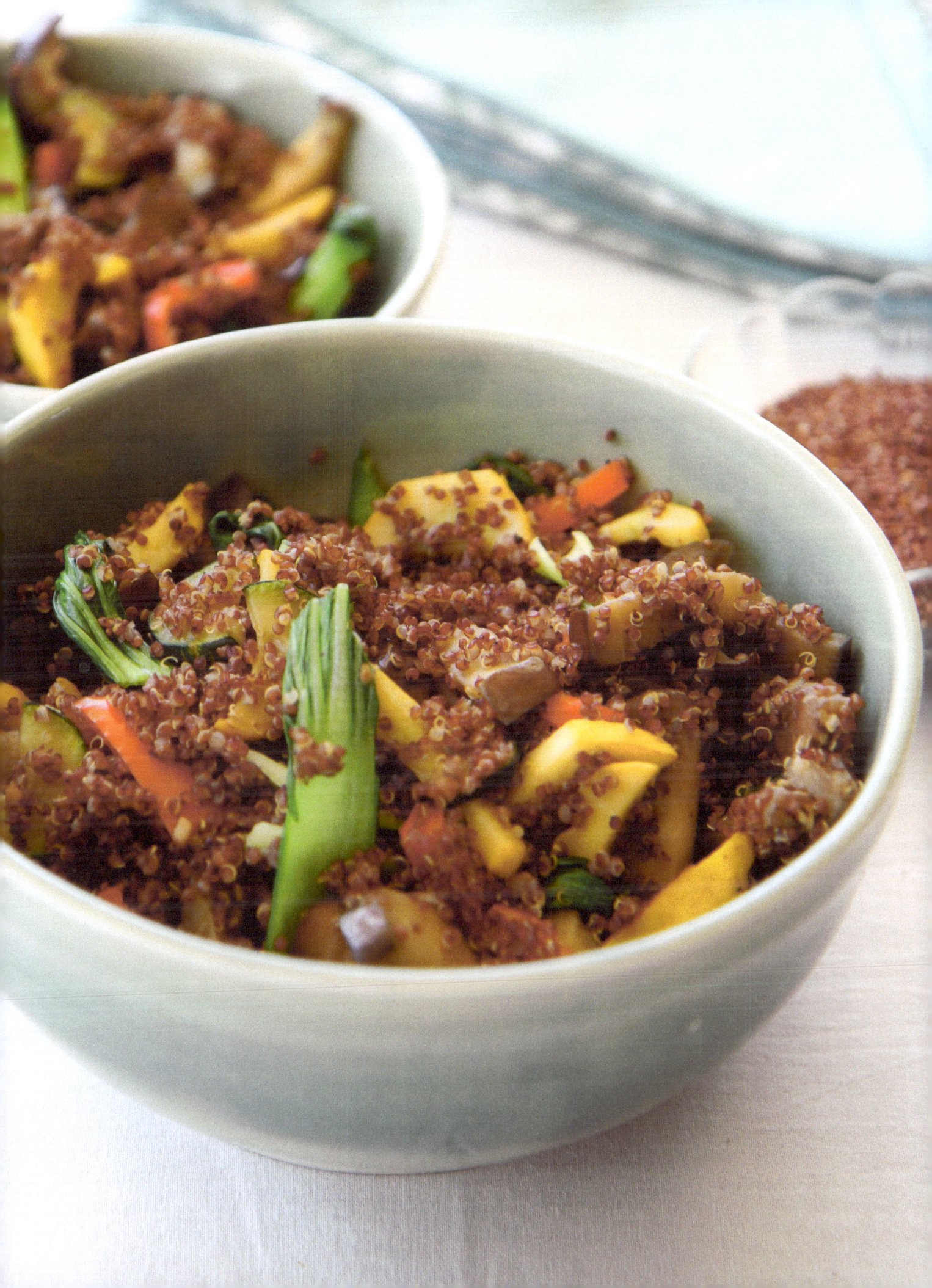

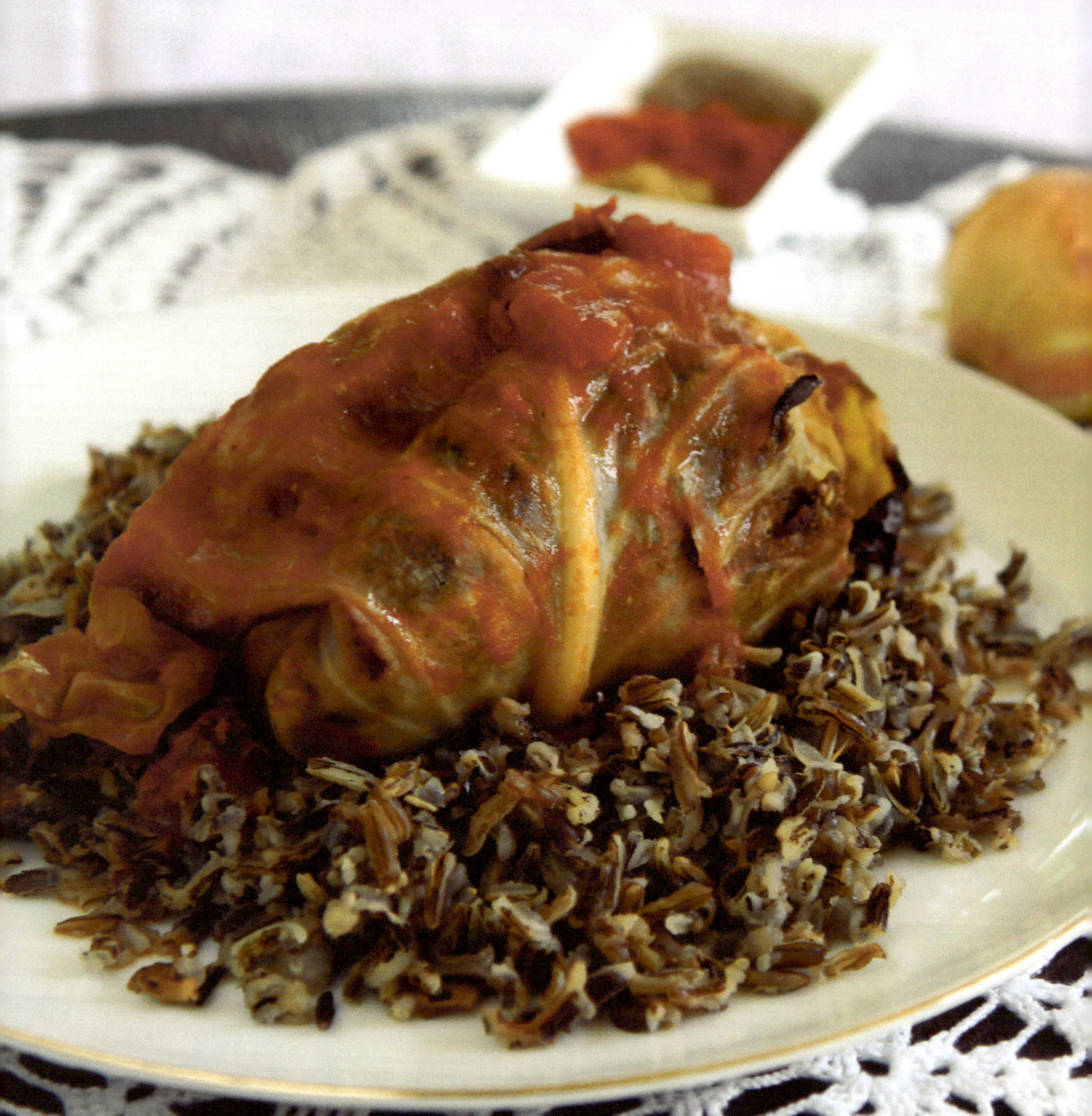

cabbage leaf hot pot

Serves 3-4 people SF

INGREDIENTS

- 5-6 large cabbage leaves (full)
- 180g packet Osem Falafel mix
- 3 ½ cups filtered water
- 400g tomatoes, diced
- 1 cup slivered almonds
- 1 cup wild rice

To make the cabbage leaves easier to remove, steam whole cabbage for a few minutes before taking leaves off.

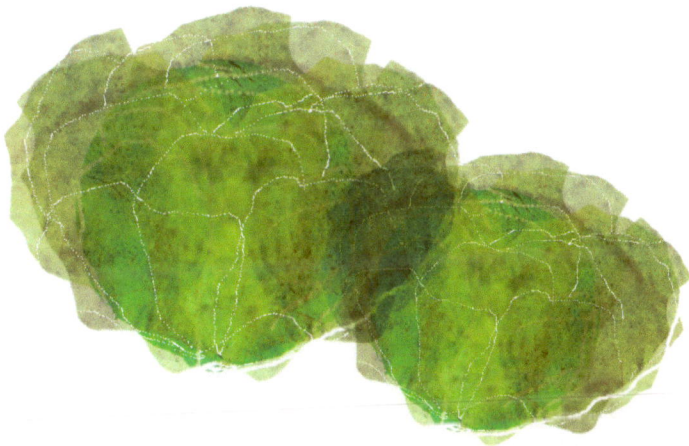

METHOD

- Preheat oven to 200°C (390°F)
- Cook wild rice and 2 cups filtered water in saucepan until tender and white forms on edges
- Empty falafel sachet into bowl and add 1 cup filtered water
- Stir through and leave for 8 minutes to absorb water
- Steam each cabbage leaf for approximately 1 minute each in microwave or in steamer
- Combine almonds with falafel mix
- Spoon mixture onto stem area of leaf - remember to keep equal amounts for the other leaves
- Fold the left and right sides of the leaf into the stem and roll up until the end
- Place rolled up leaves into casserole dish
- Combine tomatoes with ½ cup filtered water and pour this mixture over the cabbage leaves
- Cook in medium oven 200°C (390°F) for 30-40 minutes
- Serve on a bed of cooked wild rice

A mind of the calibre of mine cannot derive its nutriment from cows. A man of my spiritual intensity does not eat corpses.
- George Bernard Shaw

chilli and coriander stir-fry

Serves 3-4 people GF SF NF

INGREDIENTS

¼ pumpkin, thinly sliced
4 yellow squash, thinly sliced
1 small purple sweet potato, thinly sliced
1 zucchini (courgette), thinly sliced
2 bunches bok choy, chopped
1 fresh chilli, diced finely
1 bunch of coriander (cilantro), diced finely
400g Borlotti beans, cooked
1 cup brown rice, medium grain
3 cups filtered water

METHOD

- Boil brown rice and water in saucepan until cooked
- Stir-fry pumpkin, squash, sweet potato and zucchini in wok until tender
- Add bok choy, chilli, coriander and Borlotti beans
- Stir-fry until cooked through
- Combine with brown rice and serve

In our relations to the animal kingdom, a duty arises which all thoughtful and compassionate minds should recognise: the duty that because we are stronger in mind than the animals, we are or ought to be their guardians and helpers, not their tyrants and oppressors; and we have no right to cause them suffering or terror.

– Annie Besant

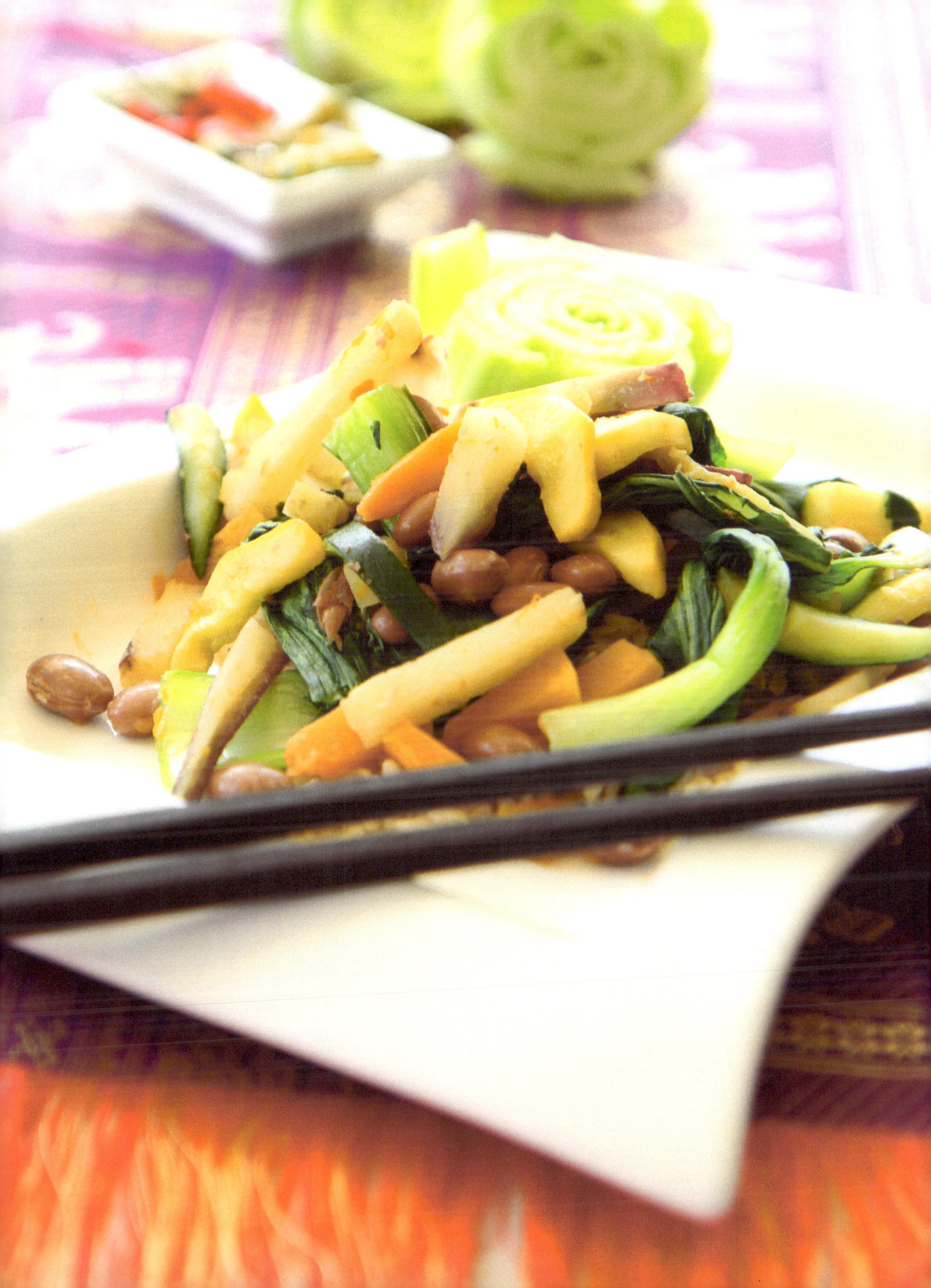

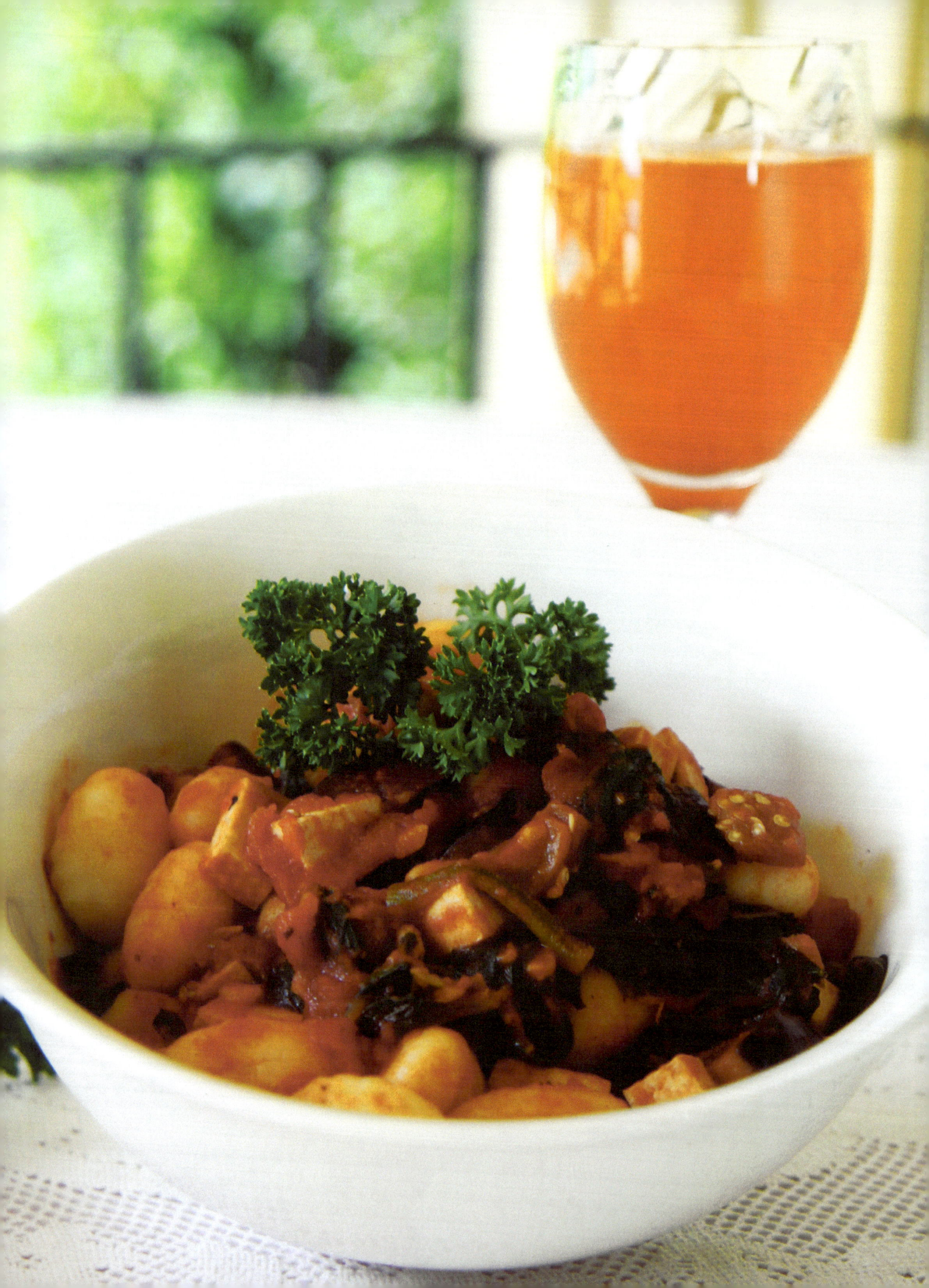

garlic gnocchi

Serves 2 people **NF**

INGREDIENTS

500g gnocchi
6 cloves of garlic, crushed
1 eggplant (aubergine), diced
8 okra, sliced thickly
¼ bunch spinach, coarsely chopped
½ pack of firm tofu (approx 150g)
5 tomatoes, diced
Extra virgin olive oil

METHOD

- Half fill a large saucepan with filtered water and bring to boil
- In a heated wok, add enough olive oil to cover the bottom, sauté the garlic cloves
- Add eggplant, okra and stir-fry until tender
- Add spinach, tofu and tomatoes and mix
- Cook gnocchi in boiling water until most of the pieces float to the surface
- Rinse gnocchi with warm water in colander then combine with vegetable mixture
- Serve with a big piece of grained garlic bread
- Serve with chopped parsley to get rid of the garlic odour

Note: this recipe originally used pumpkin gnocchi

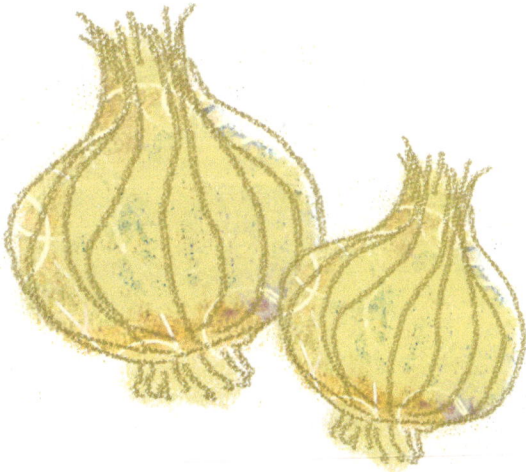

The time will come when man will look upon the murder of animals as they now look upon the murder of men.
- Leonardo da Vinci

chinese greens with eggplant

Serves 3-4 people GF NF SF

INGREDIENTS

2 eggplants (aubergine), sliced thinly
2 bunches of Chinese vegetables eg bok choy
4 garlic cloves, crushed
One inch piece of ginger, grated
¼ cup of extra virgin olive oil

METHOD

- Sauté garlic and ginger with oil in wok
- Add eggplant and stir-fry until cooked
- Add Chinese vegetables and stir through until cooked
- Serve with quinoa or brown rice mixed with LSA (linseed, sesame, almond) mix

Some of the most popular examples of Chinese greens are Chinese flowering cabbage (choi sum), Chinese broccoli (kai-lan) and Chinese chard (bok choy). Available at Chinese groceries and supermarkets.

There is the choice to love and the choice to hate,
there's the choice to inspire or the choice to turn away.
There's the choice to follow what your heart and soul attempt to voice;
but the most powerful act of all is to choose to make a choice.
- Leigh-Chantelle

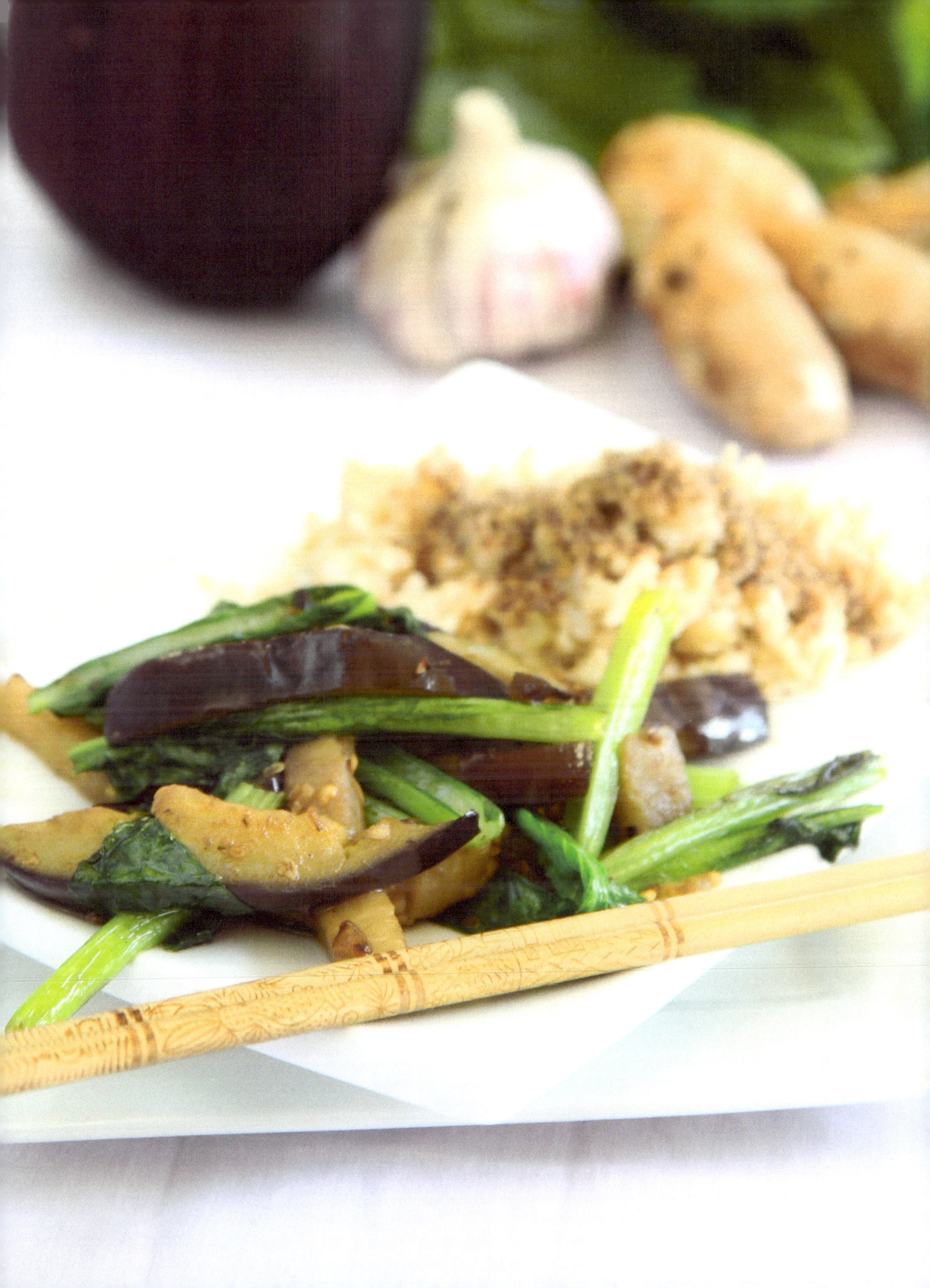

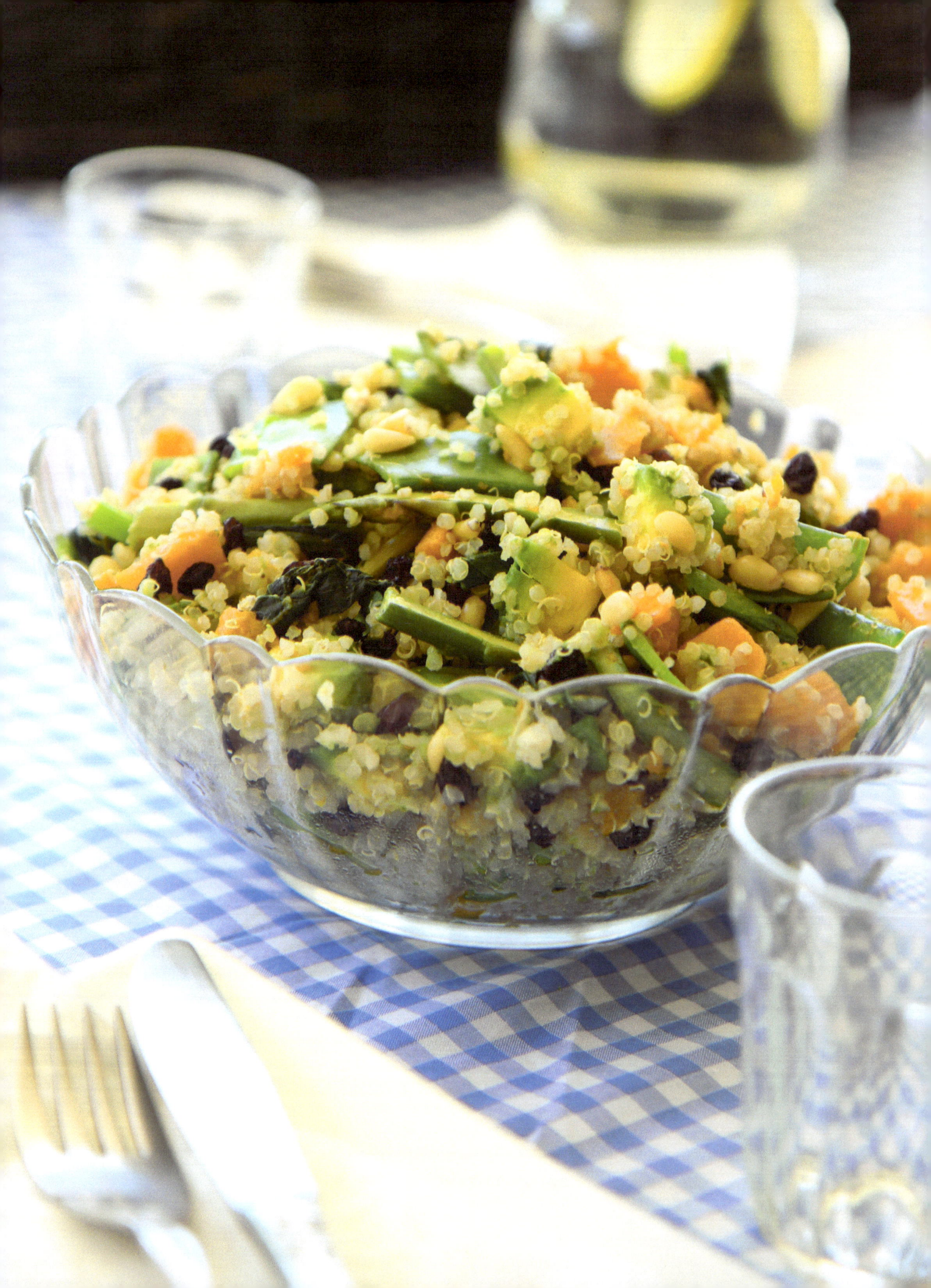

quinoa and currant salad

Serves 3-4 people **GF** **SF**

INGREDIENTS

¼ pumpkin, thinly sliced
1 asparagus bunch, cut into 1 inch pieces
2 ½ cups filtered water
½ cup snow peas, cut in half
1 bunch Chinese greens eg. Chinese broccoli, chopped
½ cup pine nuts
½ cup currants
4 avocados, diced
1 cup quinoa

METHOD

- Cook quinoa in 2 cups boiling water in saucepan or microwave until tender and a white periphery appears on the grain
- Combine cooked quinoa in a bowl with pine nuts, avocados and currants, set aside
- In a wok, stir-fry pumpkin and asparagus in ½ cup water
- Add snow peas and Chinese greens
- Stir-fry until cooked
- Cool stir-fry mix and then combine with quinoa mix
- Serve as a salad or sandwich filling

Life is life's greatest gift. Guard the life of another creature as you would your own because it is your own.
On life's scale of values, the smallest is no less precious to the creature that owns it than the largest.
- Lloyd Buggle Jr

57

millet stir-fry with bean shoots

Serves 3-4 people **GF** **SF**

INGREDIENTS

1 cup of millet
2 cups of water
2 zucchinis (courgettes), thinly sliced
¼ butternut pumpkin, thinly sliced
1 cup of green beans, cut into thirds
½ cup of LSA (linseed, sesame, almond) mix
1 cup of bean shoots
2 garlic cloves, crushed
1 onion, diced
Extra virgin olive oil

METHOD

- Bring water to boil in a medium saucepan
- Cook millet until all water is absorbed, use fork to separate grains
- Sauté garlic and onion with oil in wok
- Add zucchini, pumpkin and beans, stir-fry until cooked
- Stir through bean shoots and LSA mix
- Add cooked millet to the mix and serve

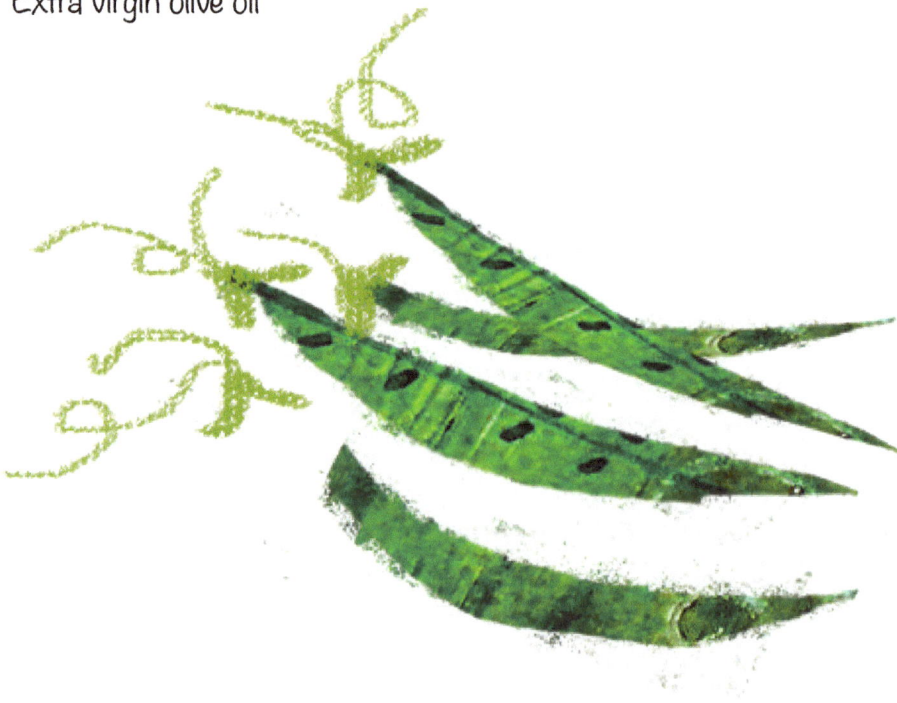

Most of our so-called reasoning consists of finding arguments for going on believing as we already do.
- James Harvey Robinson

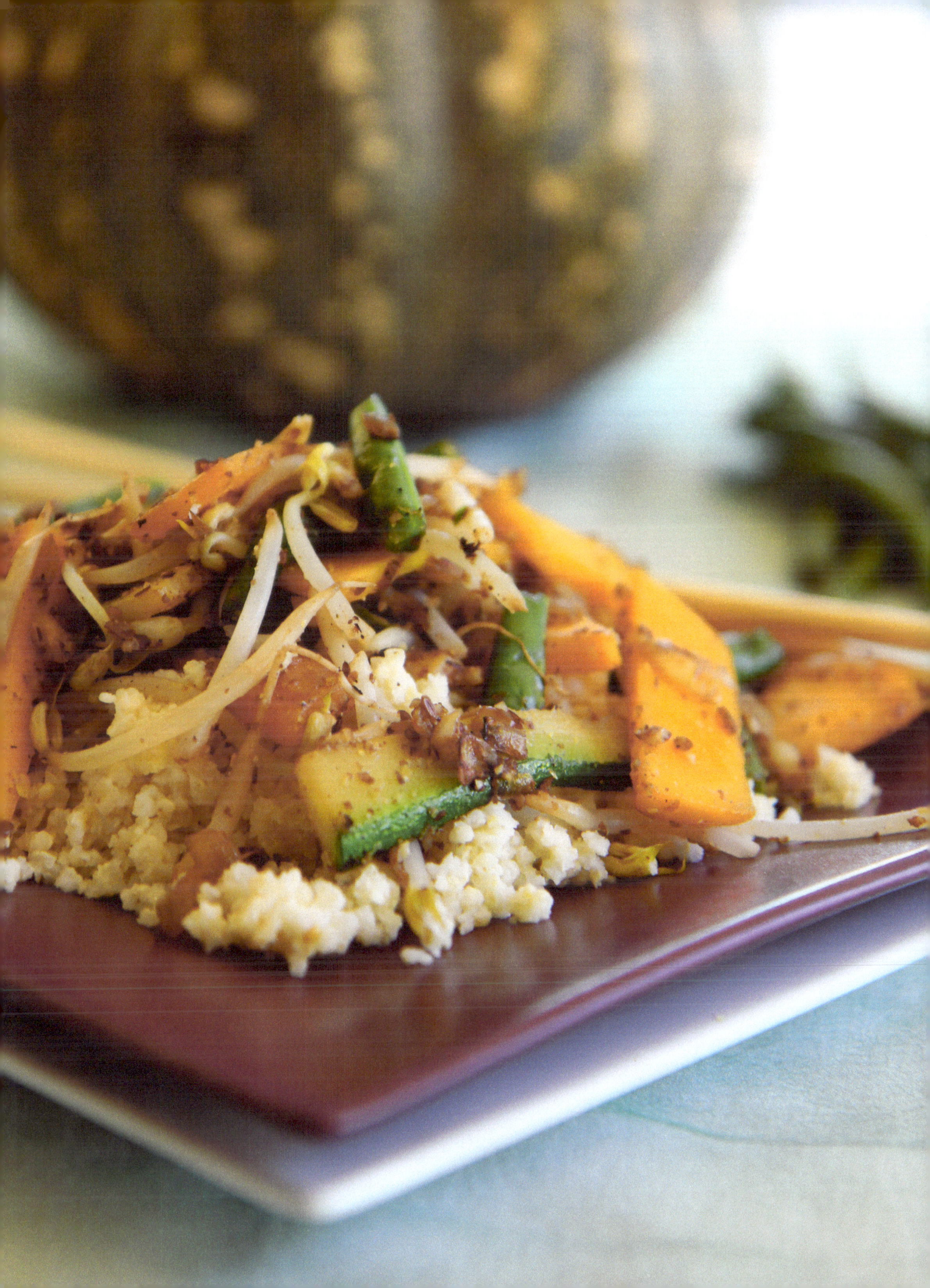

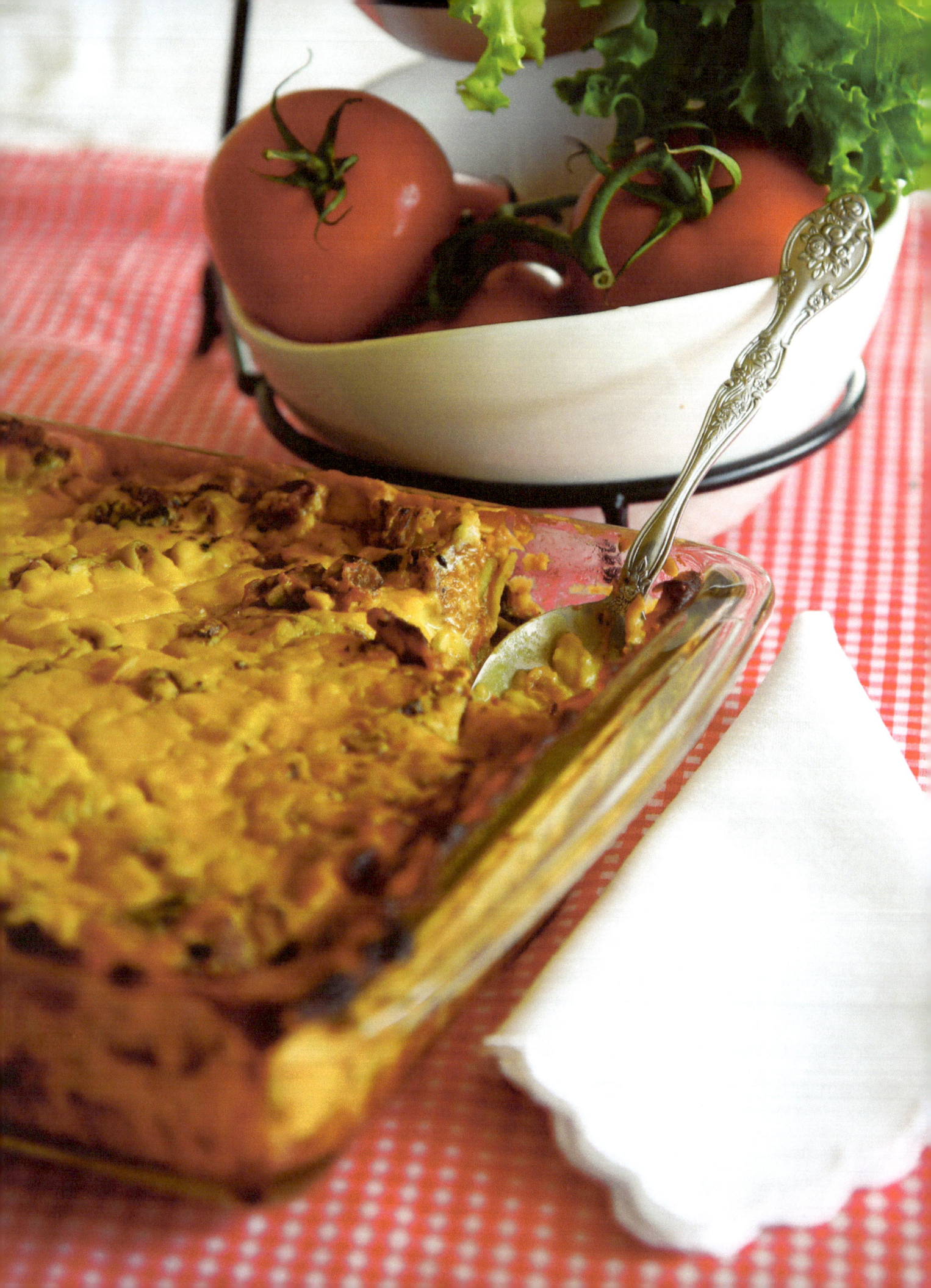

vegetable lasagne

Serves 6-8 people `GF` `SF`

INGREDIENTS

Orgran Rice and Corn Lasagne sheets (2 packs)
4 large celery stalks, cut into thick slices
¼ pumpkin, diced
4 large spinach leaves, chopped
4 tomatoes, diced
½ eggplant (aubergine), diced
1 onion, diced
2 garlic cloves, crushed
4 tbsp oregano
4 tbsp basil
Extra virgin olive oil

Cheese sauce
1 ½ cups Nutritional Yeast
½ cup besan (chickpea) flour (or another gluten-free flour)
1L (4 cups) brown rice milk (or other cruelty-free milk)
4 tbsp flax seed oil (or other oil)

METHOD

- Preheat oven to 200°C (390°F)
- Bring to boil a large saucepan of water
- Add lasagne sheets and cook until soft - approx 10 minutes
- Rinse under hot water
- Keep in cold water until required
- Sauté garlic and onion with oil in wok
- Add tomatoes, oregano and basil
- Add celery, pumpkin, eggplant and spinach
- Stir-fry until cooked
- In another saucepan, bring brown rice milk and oil to the boil
- Sift besan flour and slowly add whilst continuously stirring with a whisk
- Add nutritional yeast and stir until thick
- In a large, greased baking dish layer lasagne sheets at the bottom, half of the vegetable mix, then half of the cheese mix
- Continue with another layer of lasagne sheets, then vegetables and finish off with the remaining cheese mix
- Cook in oven at 200°C (390°F) for 15-20 minutes
- Serve warm with a salad or rye bread

Being vegan is a statement to the whole world, no matter who listens, that I am a person who cares.
- Daharja

61

polenta cakes with stir-fried vegetables

Serves 3-4 people **GF**

INGREDIENTS

1 cup polenta (cornmeal/semolina)
2 cups soymilk
10 figs, diced
10 walnuts, diced
1 onion, diced
2 garlic cloves, crushed
1 eggplant (aubergine), diced
4 spinach leaves, coarsely chopped
1 cup of beans, cut into small pieces
1 zucchini (courgette), diced
4 tomatoes, diced
Extra virgin olive oil

METHOD

- Cook polenta and 1 cup of soymilk in the microwave in 30 second successions, mixing each time
- Gradually add the remaining soymilk, continuing to mix until there is no liquid and the mixture seems to have expanded
- Mix in the walnuts and figs to the polenta mixture
- Spoon into small soufflé bowls or ramekins to set
- In heated wok, add approximately 2 tablespoons of olive oil, when heated sauté the onion and garlic
- Stir-fry eggplant, beans and zucchini in the wok
- Add tomatoes and spinach when almost complete
- To serve place serving dish on top of soufflé bowls and tip over
- Add stir-fried vegetables onto the side of the polenta cakes and serve

The greatness of a nation and its moral progress can be judged by the way its animals are treated.
- Mohandas Gahdhi

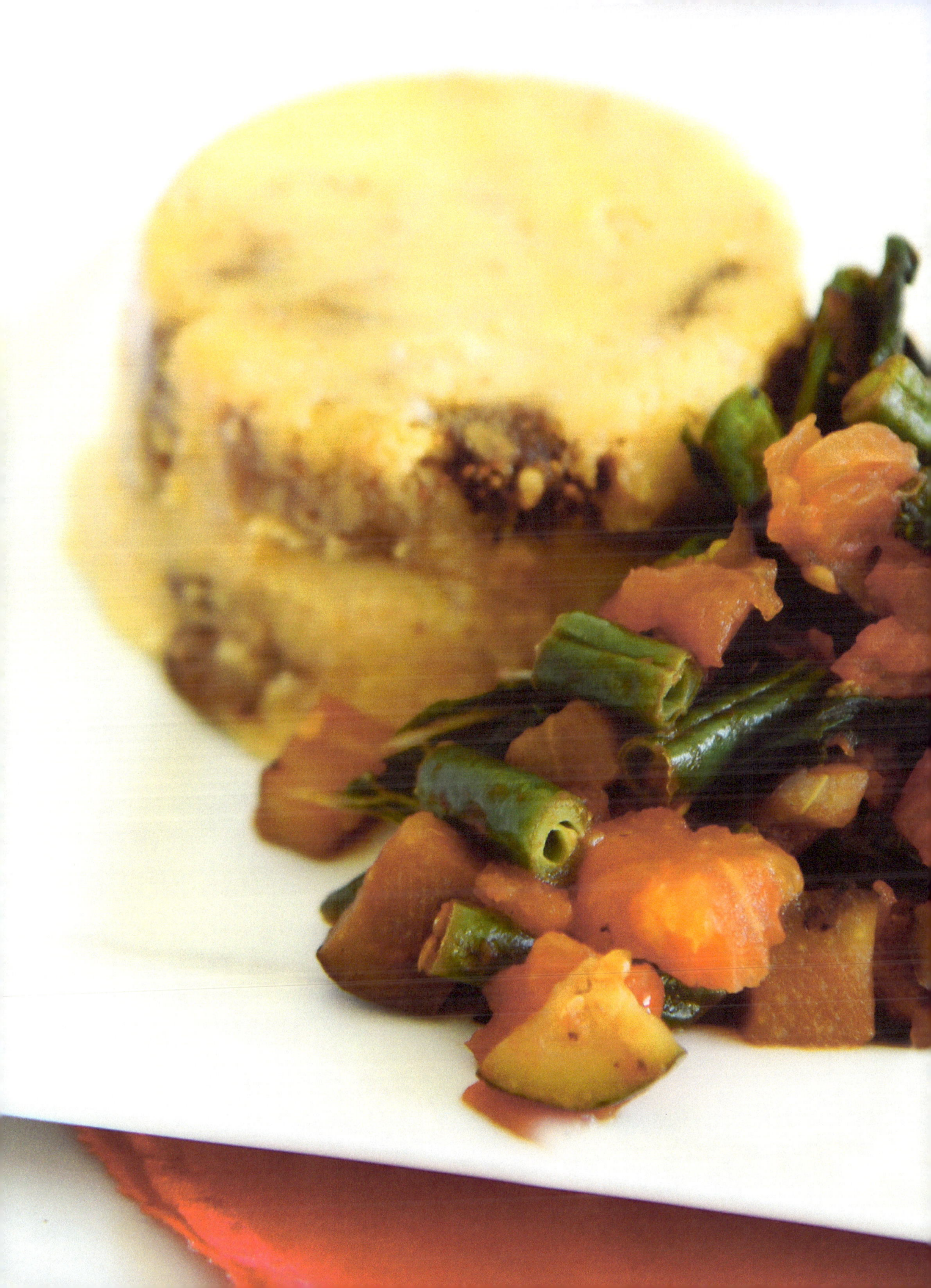

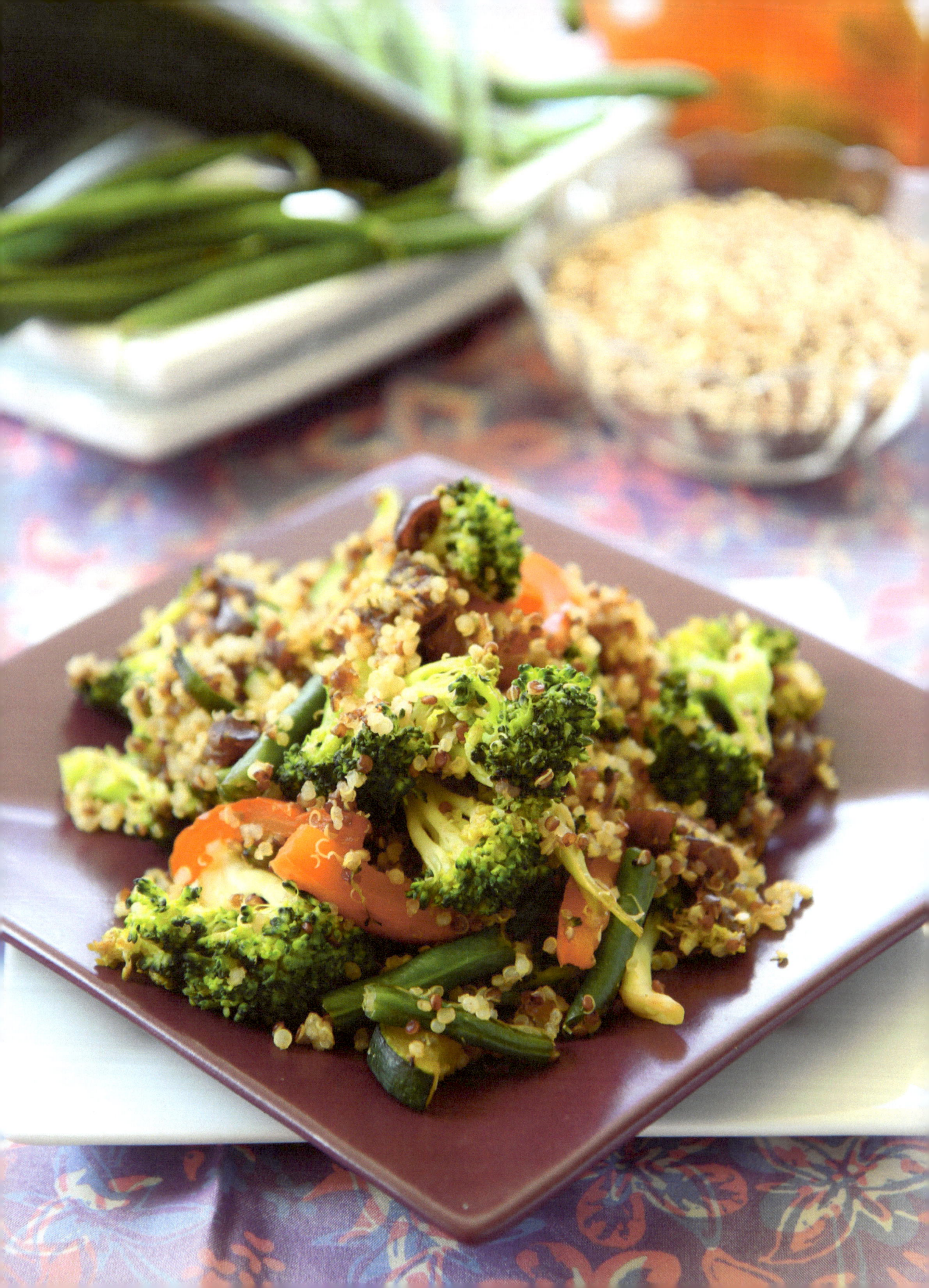

quinoa and dates stir-fry

Serves 3-4 people `GF` `NF` `SF`

INGREDIENTS

½ cup of (white) quinoa
½ cup of red Inca quinoa
2 cups of filtered water
1 zucchini (courgette), diced
1 red capsicum (pepper), thinly sliced
1 cup of beans, sliced
1 cup of broccoli florets
1 cup of dates, chopped - check for pits

METHOD

- Boil water in medium saucepan
- Add quinoa and cook until a white ring forms around the grain
- Cook zucchini, capsicum, beans and broccoli in wok with a small amount of water
- Add dates and stir-fry until cooked
- Stir through cooked quinoa and serve

Peace is not something you wish for. It's something you make, something you do, something you are; something you give away.
- Robert Fulghum

savoury pancake wraps

Serves 4-6 people SF

INGREDIENTS

375g Orgran Buckwheat Pancake Mix
450mL filtered water
3 tbsp extra virgin olive oil (plus extra)
1 large carrot, grated

200g N.S.M. falafel mix
200mL filtered water

2 avocados, thinly sliced
Hummus
LSA (linseed, sunflower and almond) mix

Hummus is a Middle Eastern and Arabic dip made by blending cooked chickpeas, tahini, oil, lemon juice and garlic. It is delicious as a spread or a dip and is a great simple snack high in protein.

METHOD

- Combine falafel mix with 200mL water in a bowl, leave for 10 minutes
- Combine pancake mix, 450mL water, oil and carrot in another bowl; mix thoroughly
- Heat oil on frypan
- Spoon pancake mix onto frying pan, cook until bubbles form
- Flip over pancake and cook until brown
- Keep pancakes warm in oven until needed

- Form falafel mix into balls - will make approximately 8
- Fry in a small amount of oil, press down onto frying pan - no need to deep fry, just a small amount of oil is required to prevent sticking
- Flip falafel onto other side, fry until brown

- When ready to serve meal, spread pancake with hummus
- Sprinkle with LSA mix and crumble falafel onto pancake
- Place avocado on top and roll up pancake
- Left over mix can be used to make pikelets for a healthy snack

The love for all living creatures is the most noble attribute of man.
- Charles Darwin

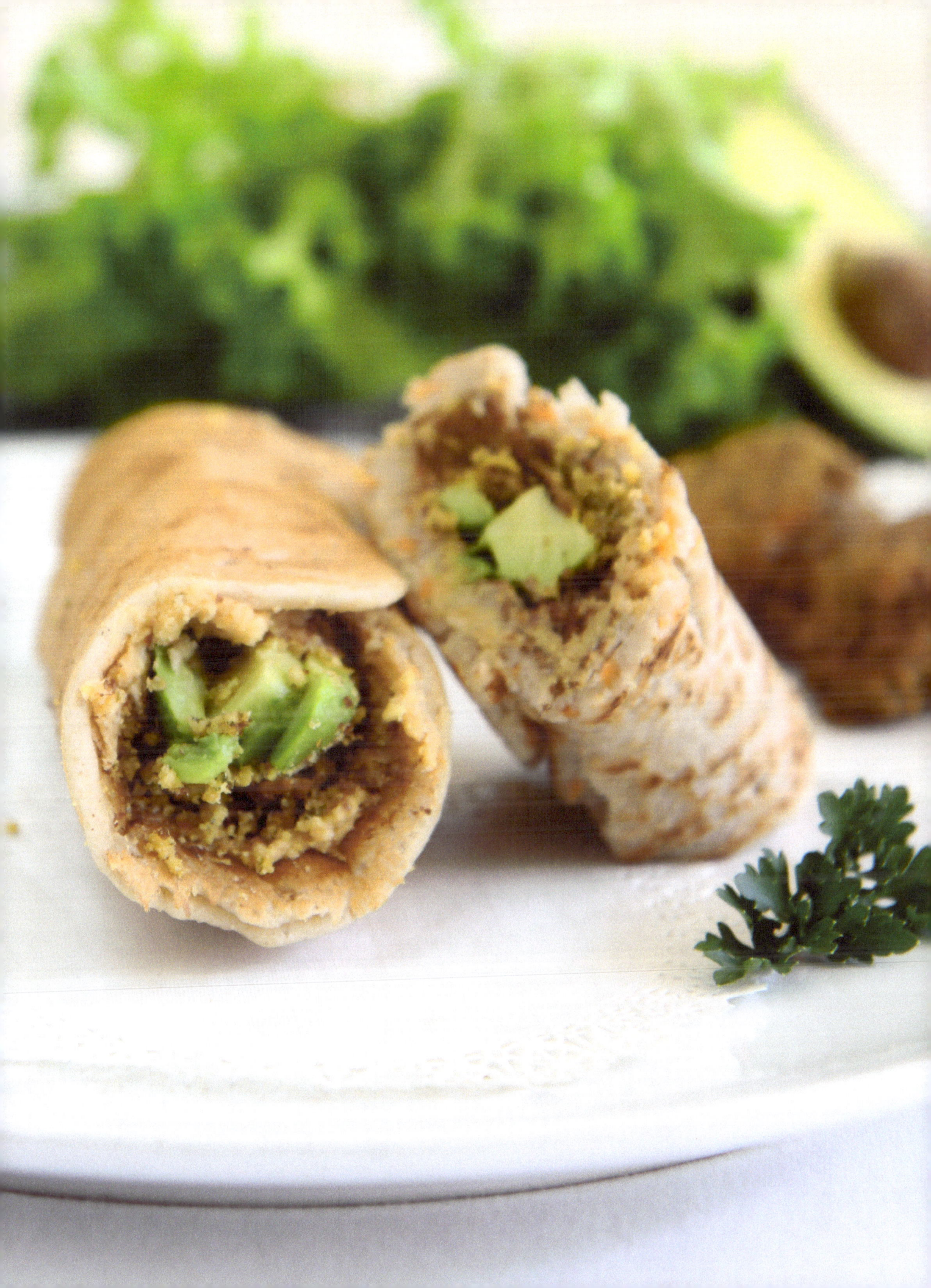

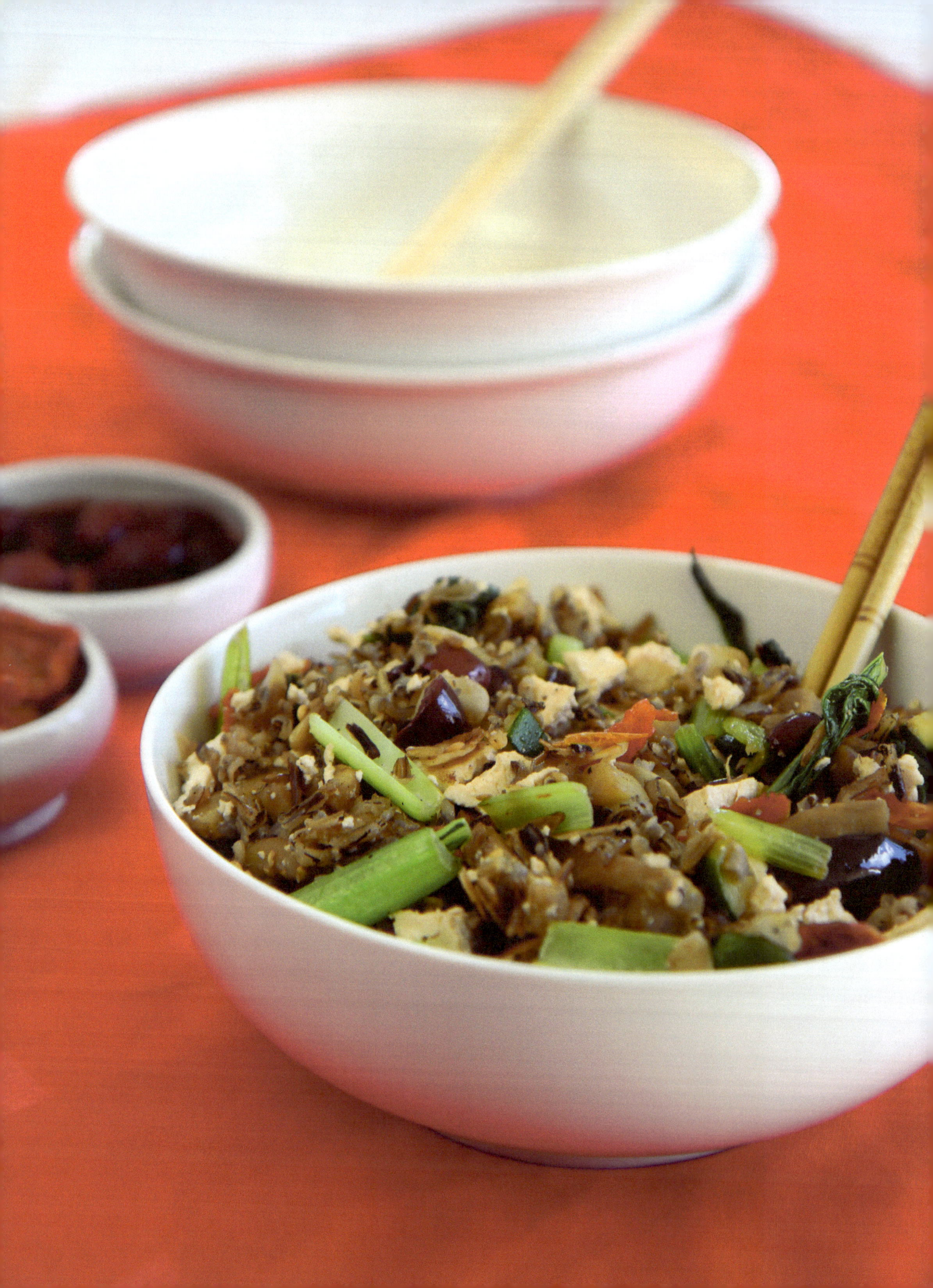

Wild rice and mediterranean vegetables

Serves 4-6 people **GF**

INGREDIENTS

1 cup wild rice
1 cup long grain brown rice
4 cups filtered water
2 garlic cloves, crushed
1 zucchini (courgette), diced
½ eggplant (aubergine), thinly sliced
2 bunches Chinese greens eg Chinese broccoli, chopped
1 cup olives, diced and pitted if needed
1 cup sun-dried tomatoes
1 cup almond flakes
375g silken tofu, crumbled

METHOD

- Cook wild and brown rice in boiling water until tender (approx 20 minutes)
- Sauté garlic in wok
- Add eggplant and zucchini, stir-fry until cooked
- Add Chinese greens, cook until soft
- Add sun-dried tomatoes, olives, tofu and almond flakes, mix well
- Combine with rice mixture

Wild rice is an aquatic grain that grows in regions in North America and Asia. Wild rice has a beautiful dark colour and texture that takes less time to cook than brown rice.
It can be used instead of brown rice, or a combination of the two and can be purchased from health food stores.

Until we have the courage to recognise cruelty for what it is – whether its victim is human or animal – we cannot expect things to be much better in this world... We cannot have peace among men whose hearts delight in killing any living creature. By every act that glorifies or even tolerates such moronic delight in killing we set back the progress of humanity.
- Rachel Carson

pumpkin and asparagus tofu

Serves 3-4 people GF

INGREDIENTS

¼ pumpkin, diced in small pieces
300g tofu, cut into large strips
2 asparagus bunches, cut length-ways in quarters
Handful of coriander (cilantro), roughly chopped
1 cup of pine nuts

METHOD

- Cook pumpkin in wok with a small amount of water
- Add coriander and asparagus, stir fry
- Add tofu and pine nuts, stir fry until cooked
- Serve with brown rice or as is

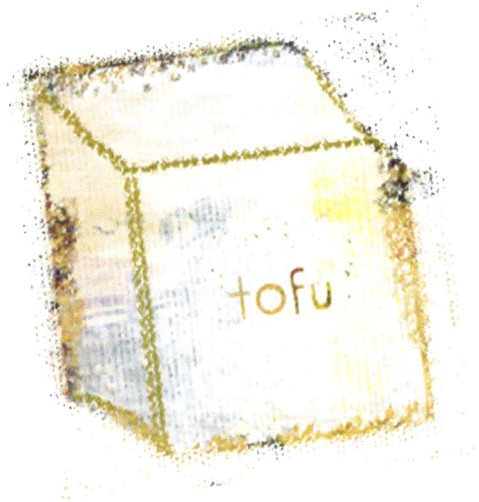

Do all the good you can, by all the means you can, in all the ways you can, in all the places you can, at all the times you can, to all the people you can, as long as ever you can.
- John Wesley

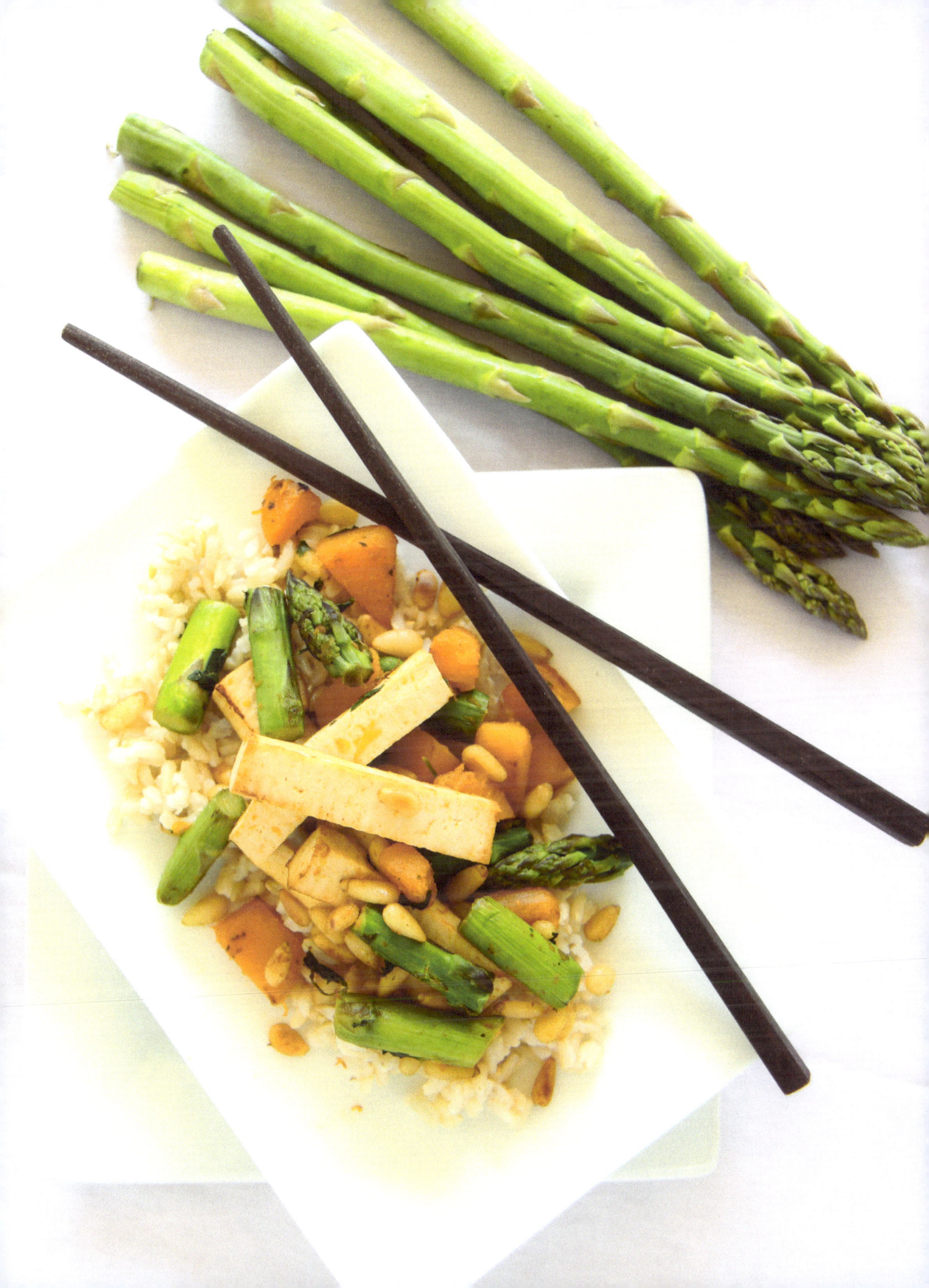

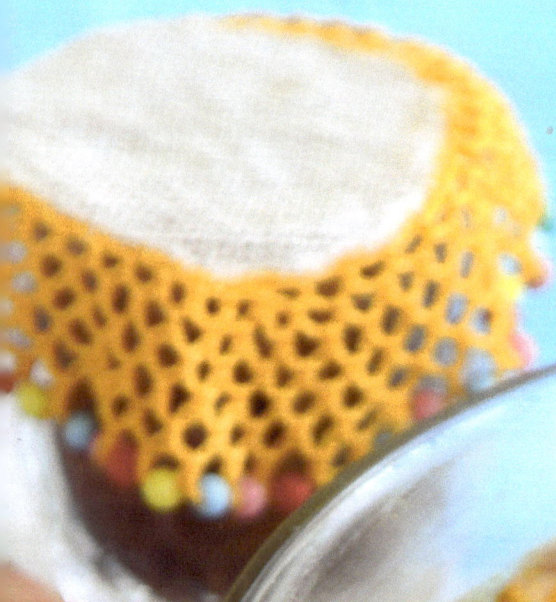

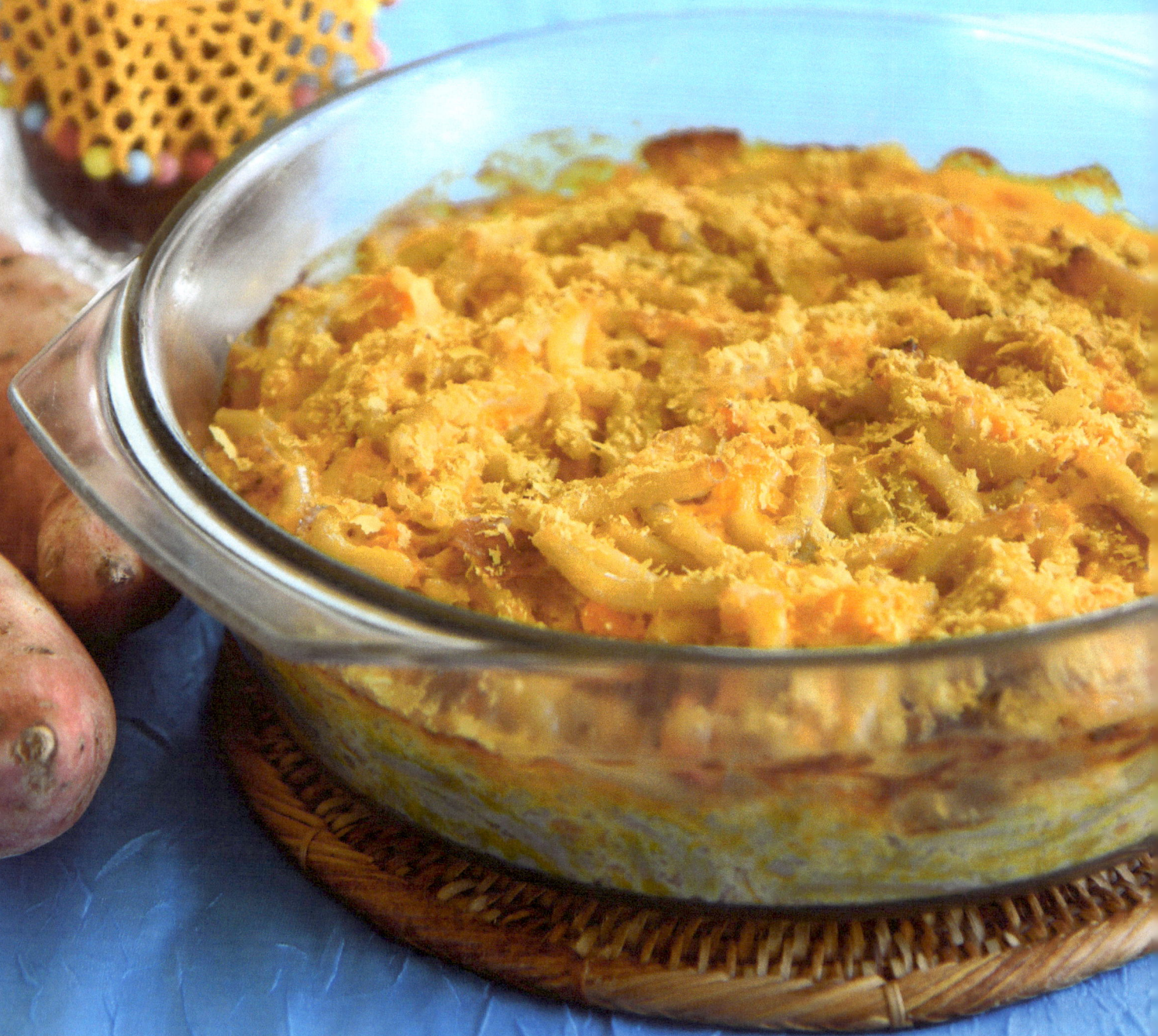

vegetable pasta bake

Serves 4-6 people GF NF

INGREDIENTS

1 sweet potato, diced
¼ pumpkin, diced
350g Berconia brown rice macaroni
Filtered water
250g soy cream cheese
Nutritional yeast

METHOD

- Cook macaroni and filtered water in saucepan until tender
- Cook sweet potato and pumpkin together in a separate saucepan or wok
- Mash together
- Combine with soy cream cheese
- Add macaroni and stir through
- Sprinkle with nutritional yeast
- Serve with warm rye bread

Nutritional Yeast is from an organism grown on molasses and deactivated. This inactive form doesn't make things grow like Brewer's yeast, as it has no leavening ability. Also known as Noosh, Hippy Dust and Savoury Yeast. Some brands have vitamin B12 added.

The thinking man must oppose all cruel customs no matter how deeply rooted in tradition and surrounded by halo. When we have a choice, we must avoid bringing torment and injury into the life of another, even the lowliest creature; to do so is to renounce our manhood and shoulder a guilt which nothing justifies.
- Dr. Albert Schweizer

tempeh stir-fry

Serves 3-4 people GF NF

INGREDIENTS

2 bunches of Chinese greens eg bok choy
4 squash, thinly sliced
1 red capsicum (pepper), thinly sliced
1 green capsicum (pepper), thinly sliced
½ sweet potato, thinly sliced
1 bunch of asparagus, thinly sliced
200g tempeh, sliced
1 cup of soy or brown rice milk

METHOD

- Stir-fry sweet potato in wok with a small amount of water
- Add capsicum, squash, asparagus and stir-fry
- Mix through milk and bring to boil
- Add tempeh and Chinese greens - stir through
- Serve with brown rice if desired

Tempeh is a great source of protein and calcium, traditionally made in Indonesia. It is made by fermenting cooked soybeans and moulding into a patty. The tempeh flavour is nutty and has a unique flavour on its own.

Never apologise for showing feelings. When you do you apologise for the truth.
- Benjamin Disraeli

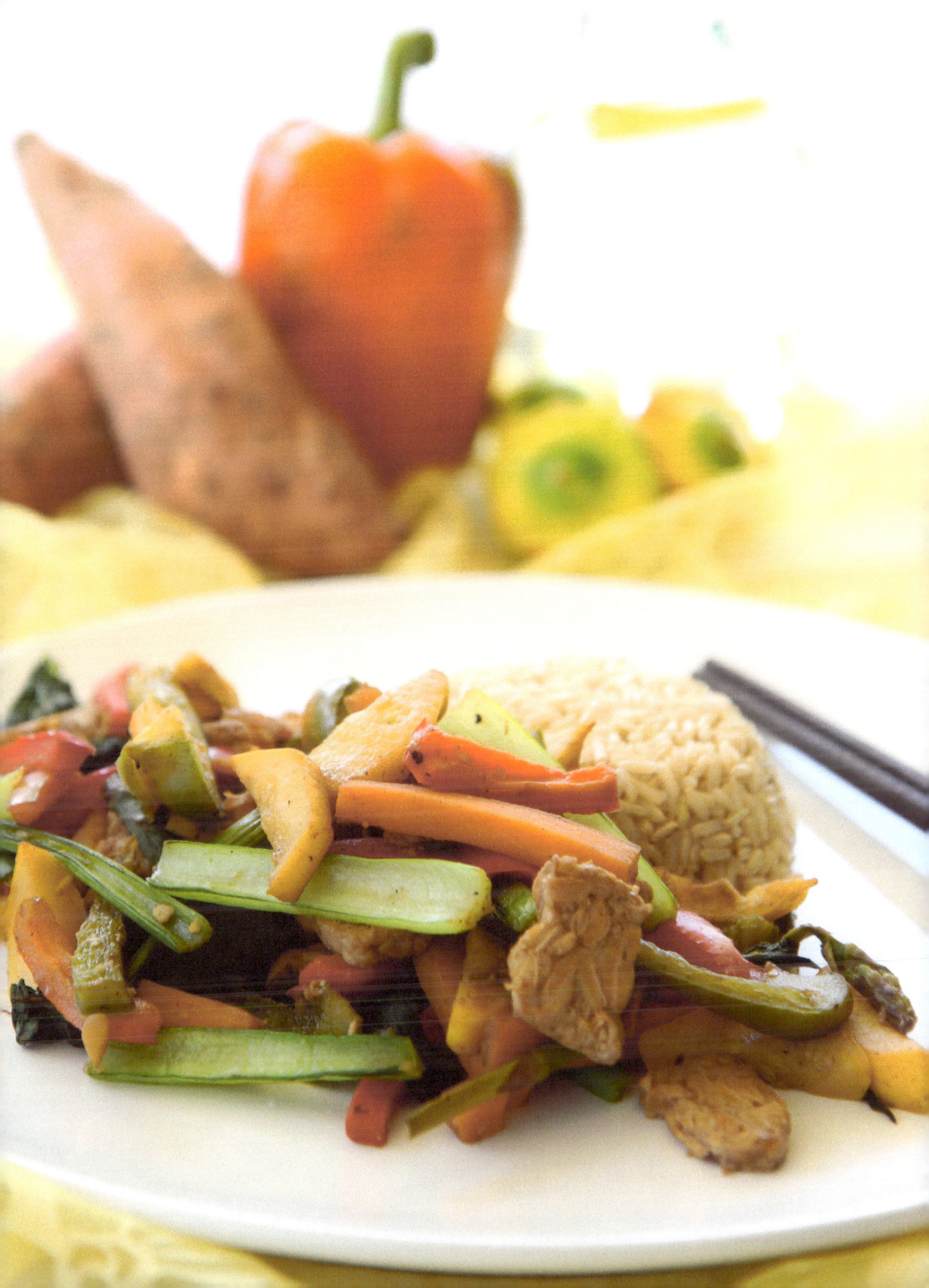

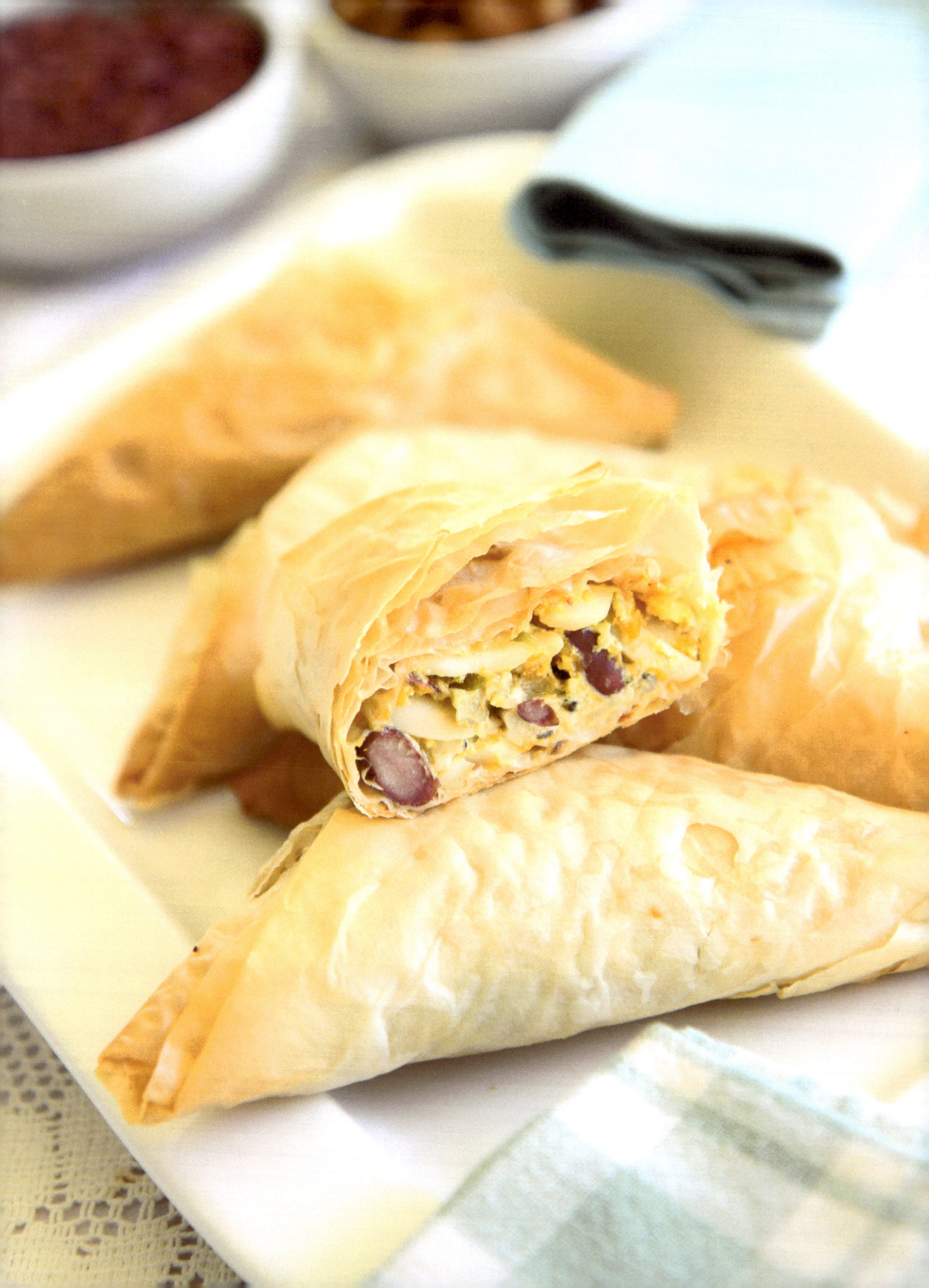

vegetable pasties

Serves 4-6 people

INGREDIENTS

2 zucchini (courgette), grated
¼ pumpkin, grated
½ eggplant (aubergine), thinly sliced
400g red kidney beans, cooked
250g soy cream cheese
1 cup slivered almonds
1 tblsp cracked black pepper
1 packet Antoniou filo pastry
Extra virgin olive oil

METHOD

- Preheat oven to 200°C (390°F)
- Cook eggplant, pumpkin and zucchini in wok
- Add almonds, cheese, beans and pepper and mix well
- Cool down mixture
- Oil filo pastry sheets as per diagram
- Spoon filling onto edge of sheet
- Fold sheet as per diagram, oil outside
- Cook in medium oven 200°C (390°F) for 30-40 minutes or until golden
- Serve as a main meal or as an appetiser
- Makes approximately 16 pasties

how to fold:

1. **fold in half** — oil

2. **fold in half again** — oil

3. **spoon on filling**

fold diagonally brushwith oil

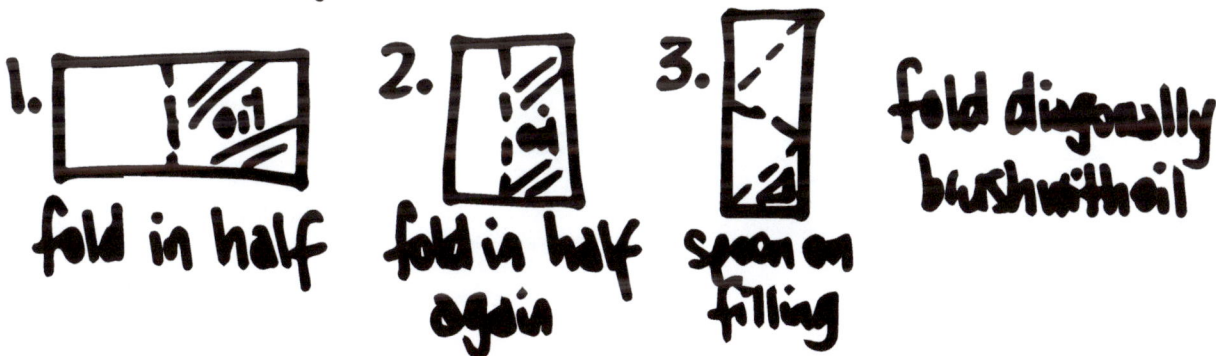

A man can live and be healthy without killing animals for food; therefore, if he eats meat he participates in taking animal life merely for the sake of his appetite. And to act so is immoral.

- Leo Tolstoy

chilli quinoa

Serves 3-4 people `GF` `NF` `SF`

INGREDIENTS

1 broccoli bunch, separated into flowerettes
2 zucchini (courgette), thinly sliced lengthways
1 red capsicum (pepper), thinly sliced
¼ pumpkin, thinly sliced
2 bunches Chinese broccoli (or another Chinese green)
400g red kidney beans, cooked
1 cup quinoa
2 cups filtered water
1 red chilli, finely chopped

METHOD

- Cook quinoa and water in saucepan until white rim forms on the periphery of the grain
- Stir-fry broccoli, zucchini, capsicum, pumpkin and chilli until cooked
- Add Chinese broccoli and red kidney beans
- Combine cooked quinoa with vegetables and serve

If (man) is not to stifle his human feelings, he must practice kindness towards animals, for he who is cruel to animals becomes hard also in his dealings with men. We can judge the heart of a man by his treatment of animals.
– Immanuel Kant

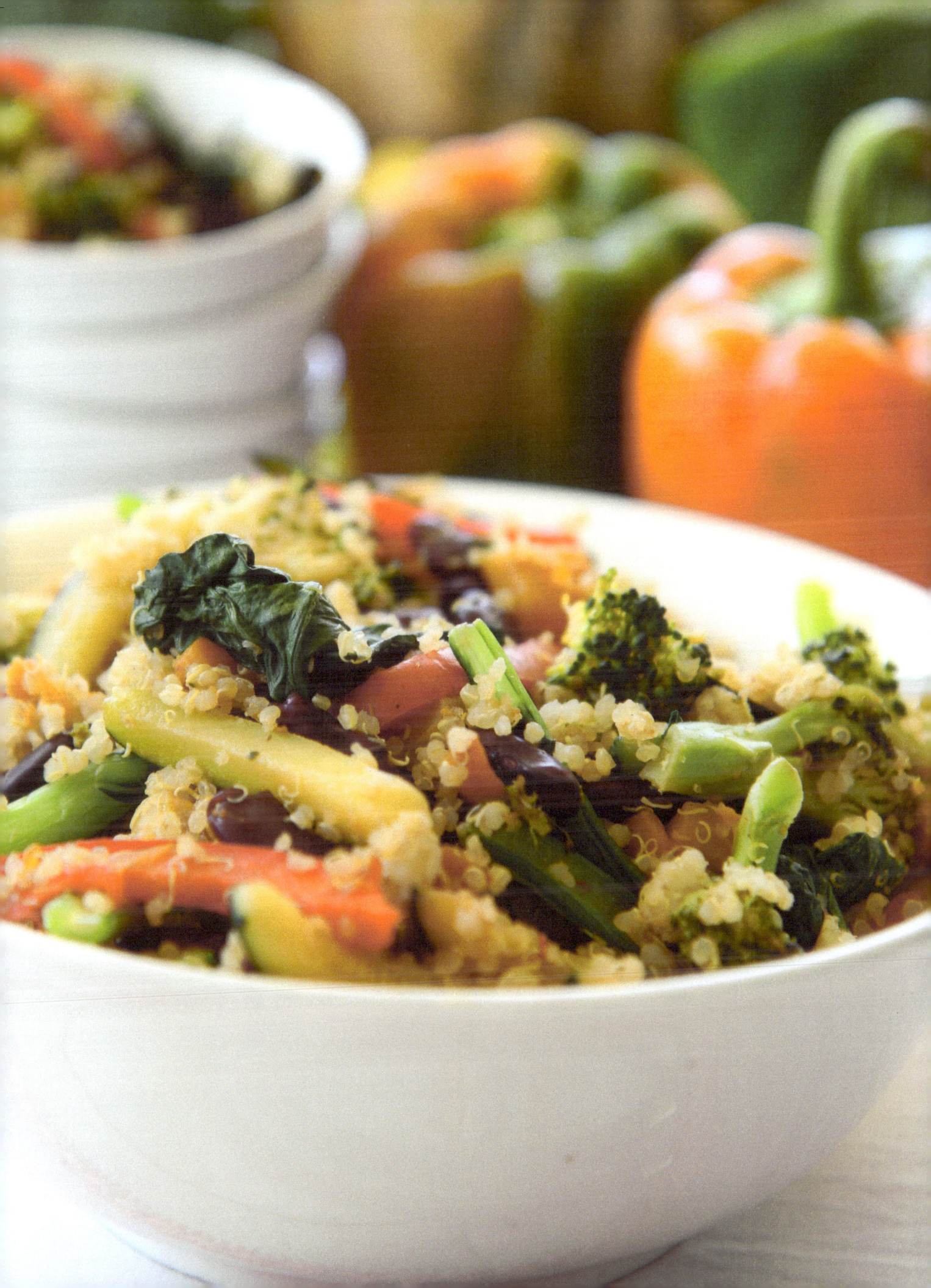

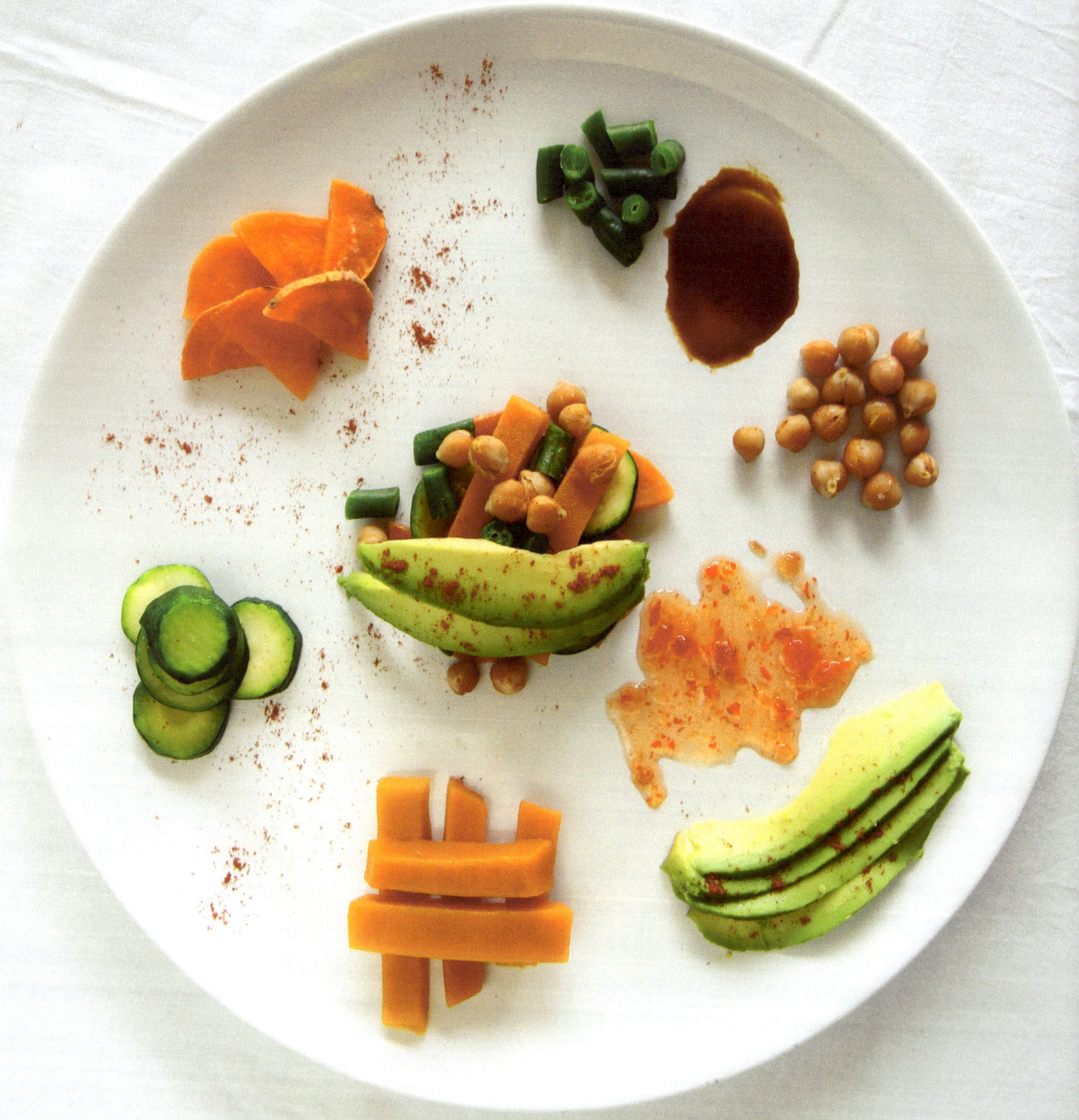

vegetable and chickped salad

Serves 2-4 people GF NF SF

INGREDIENTS

1 sweet potato, cut in semi-circles
2 zucchinis (courgette), cut into circles
¼ pumpkin, cut into sticks
1 cup of beans, cut in small pieces
1 avocado, thinly sliced
400g chickpeas, cooked
Sweet chilli sauce
Cayenne pepper

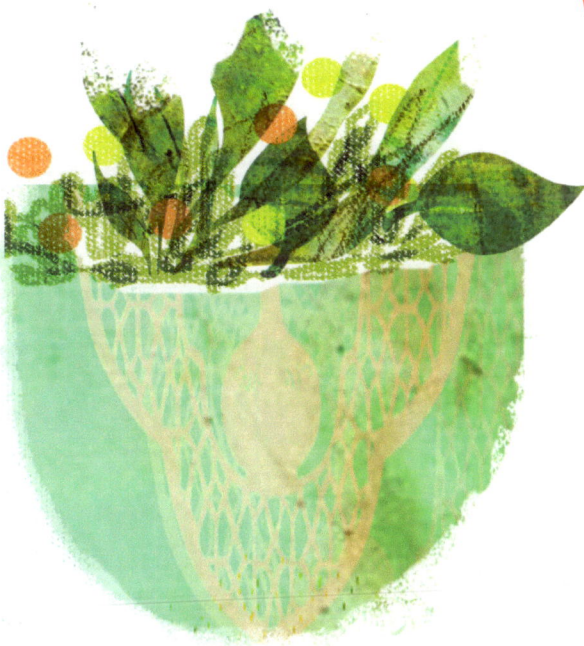

METHOD

- Cook vegetables separately in microwave or pot on stove, then drain
- Layer sweet potato in a circle right in the middle of your plate and drizzle with sweet chilli sauce
- Position the zucchini circles on top
- Place pumpkin across with the beans and chickpeas between each pumpkin piece
- Fan avocado slice on top of salad and sprinkle with cayenne pepper
- Decoratively circle the main salad with separate piles of the vegetables if making one large serving dish
- Sprinkle with cayenne pepper and a dash of sweet chilli sauce
- Serve as a main meal with brown rice or as a salad

Chickpeas (Garbanzo beans) are a great source of calcium and protein and are one of the most delicious of the pulses. Beans need to be soaked overnight and then cooked or you can buy cans that are already cooked - just make sure that you rinse well before using.

Facts do not cease to exist because they are ignored.
- A. Huxley

81

Wild rice with eggplant

Serves 4-6 people GF NF SF

INGREDIENTS

1 ½ cups of wild rice
4 cups of water
1 eggplant (aubergine), sliced
2 squash, thinly sliced
¼ pumpkin, diced
4 tomatoes, diced
400g red kidney beans, cooked
Extra virgin olive oil
1 onion, diced
2 garlic cloves, crushed
4 tbsp basil
4 tbsp oregano
2 tbsp cracked black pepper

METHOD

- Bring water to boil in a large saucepan
- Cook wild rice - approximately 30 mins
- Sauté garlic and onion with oil in wok
- Add tomatoes, basil, pepper and oregano
- Add pumpkin, squash and eggplant; stir-fry until cooked
- Mix through red kidney beans and cooked rice
- Serve with rye bread

A human being is a part of a whole, called by us universe, a part limited in time and space. He experiences himself, his thoughts and feelings as something separated from the rest... a kind of optical delusion of his consciousness. This delusion is a kind of prison for us, restricting us to our personal desires and to affection for a few persons nearest to us. Our task must be to free ourselves from this prison by widening our circle of compassion to embrace all living creatures and the whole of nature and its beauty.
– Albert Einstein

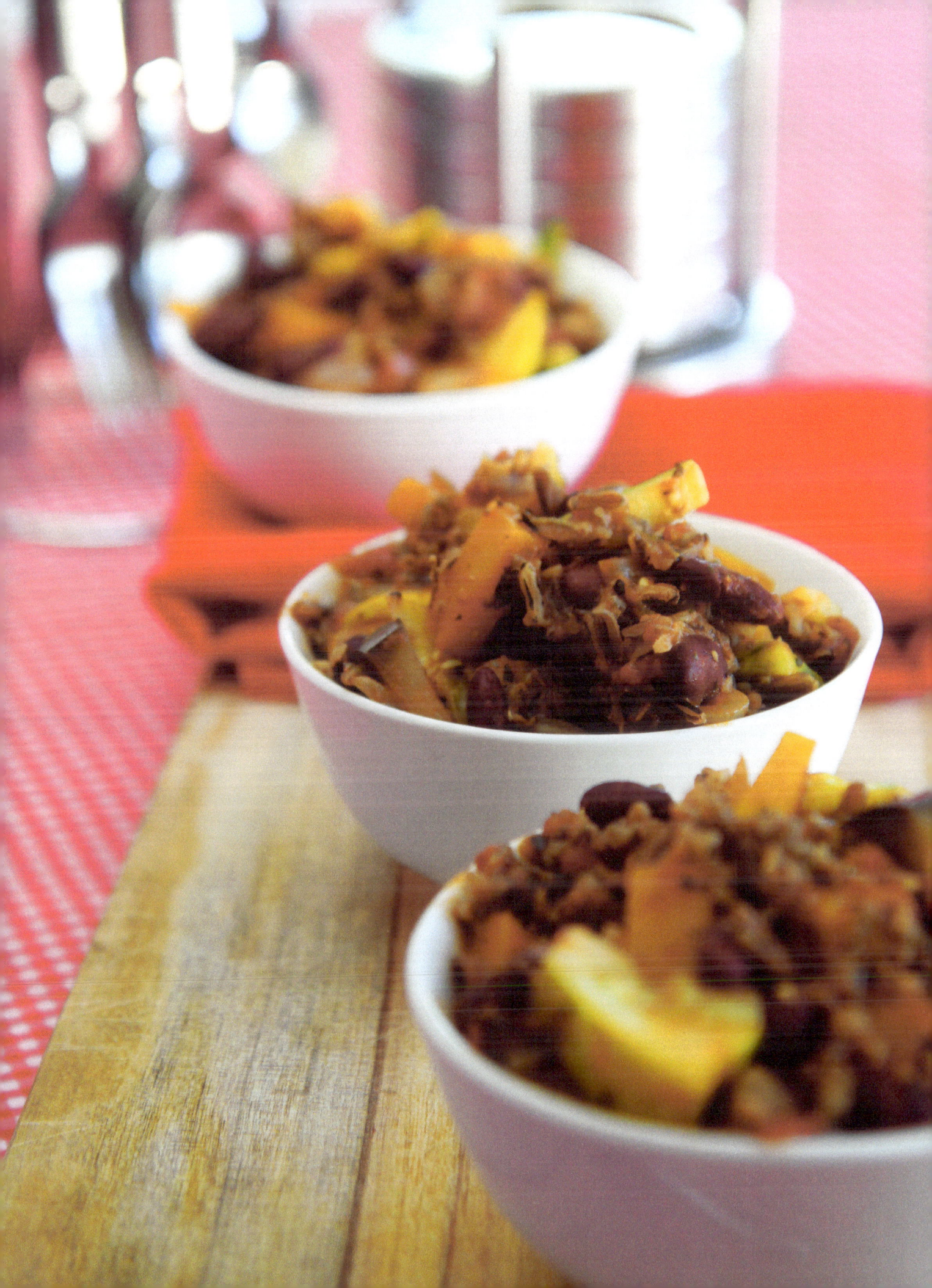

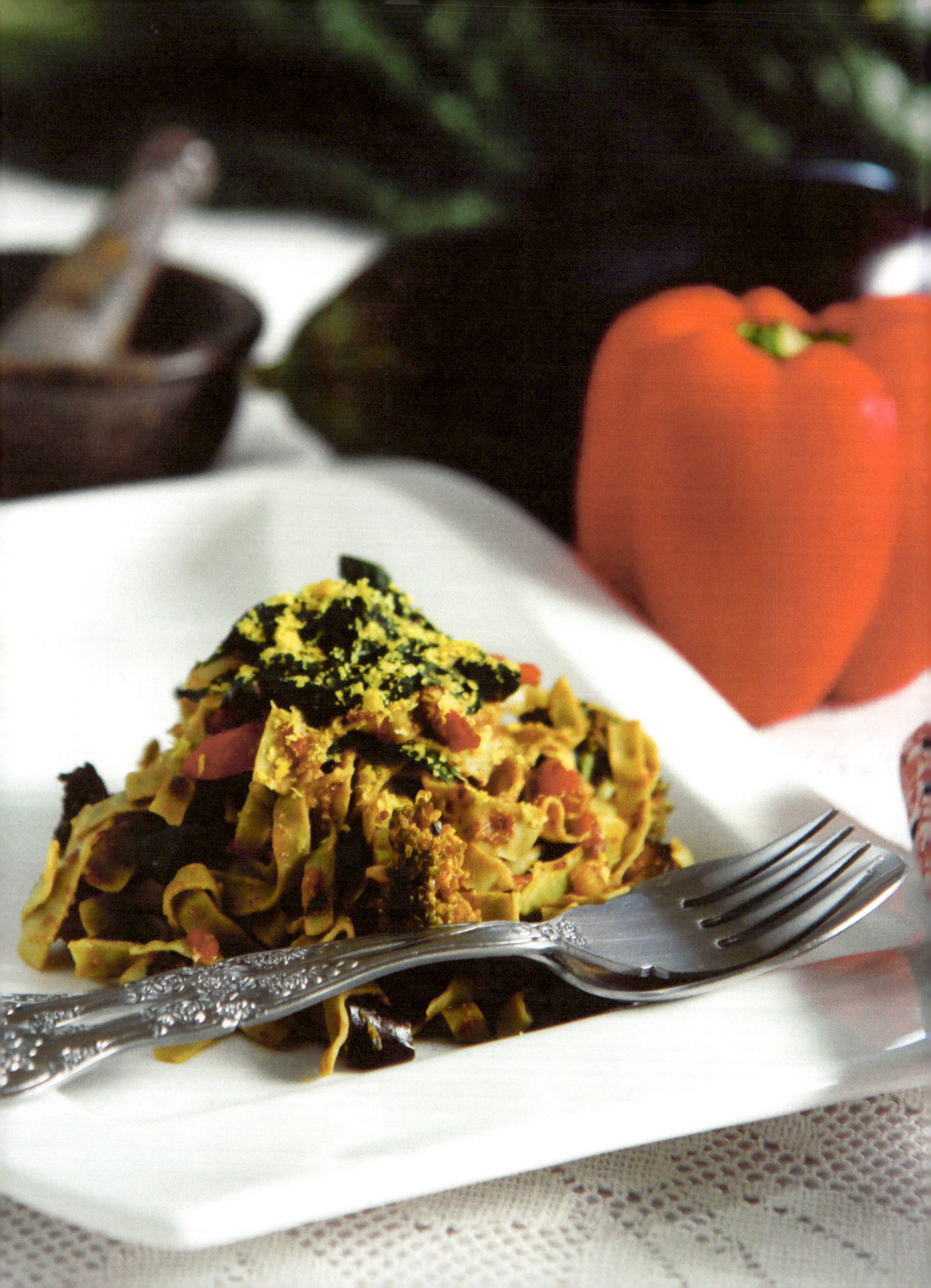

mung bean fettuccine with spinach

Serves 4-6 people GF SF

INGREDIENTS

200g Explore Asian Organic Mung Bean Fettuccine
1 eggplant (aubergine), cut into strips
1 red capsicum (pepper), cut into strips
2 zucchinis (courgettes), cut into strips
½ bunch of spinach, coarsely cut
1 cup of broccoli florets
½ cup LSA (linseed, sesame, almond) mix
4 tomatoes, diced
2 garlic cloves, crushed
Extra virgin olive oil
Oregano
Cracked black pepper
Nutritional Yeast

METHOD

- Bring a large saucepan of water to the boil
- Add fettuccine
- Continue to boil until cooked, approx 8-12 minutes
- Sauté garlic and oil in wok
- Add oregano, pepper and tomatoes
- Stir through zucchini, capsicum and broccoli, cook with wok covered
- After 5-10 minutes, add eggplant
- Add spinach, stir through until cooked
- Stir through cooked pasta and LSA mix
- Top with nutritional yeast to taste

Note: This recipe was previously known as Soybean pasta with spinach

Refrain at all times from such foods as cannot be procured without violence and oppression.
Thomas Tryon

sweet potato and pumpkin curry

Serves 4-6 people GF SF

INGREDIENTS

1 large sweet potato, diced into medium sized pieces
¼ pumpkin, diced into medium sized pieces
400mL coconut cream
1 tsp coriander (cilantro) powder
1 tsp cardamom seed powder
1 tsp cumin powder
1 cup long grain brown rice
3 cups filtered water
400g chickpeas (garbanzo beans), cooked
½ bunch silverbeet or spinach, coarsely chopped

METHOD

- Cook brown rice and water in saucepan until tender
- Combine spices and coconut cream in a container and set aside
- Stir-fry sweet potato and pumpkin for 5 minutes in wok
- Add cream and spice mix
- Turn down to medium heat and simmer for 15 minutes
- Add silverbeet or spinach and chickpeas - combine well
- Serve with rice and pappadums

Compassion is the foundation of everything positive, everything good. If you can carry the power of compassion to the marketplace and the dinner table, you can make your life really count.
- Rue McClanahan

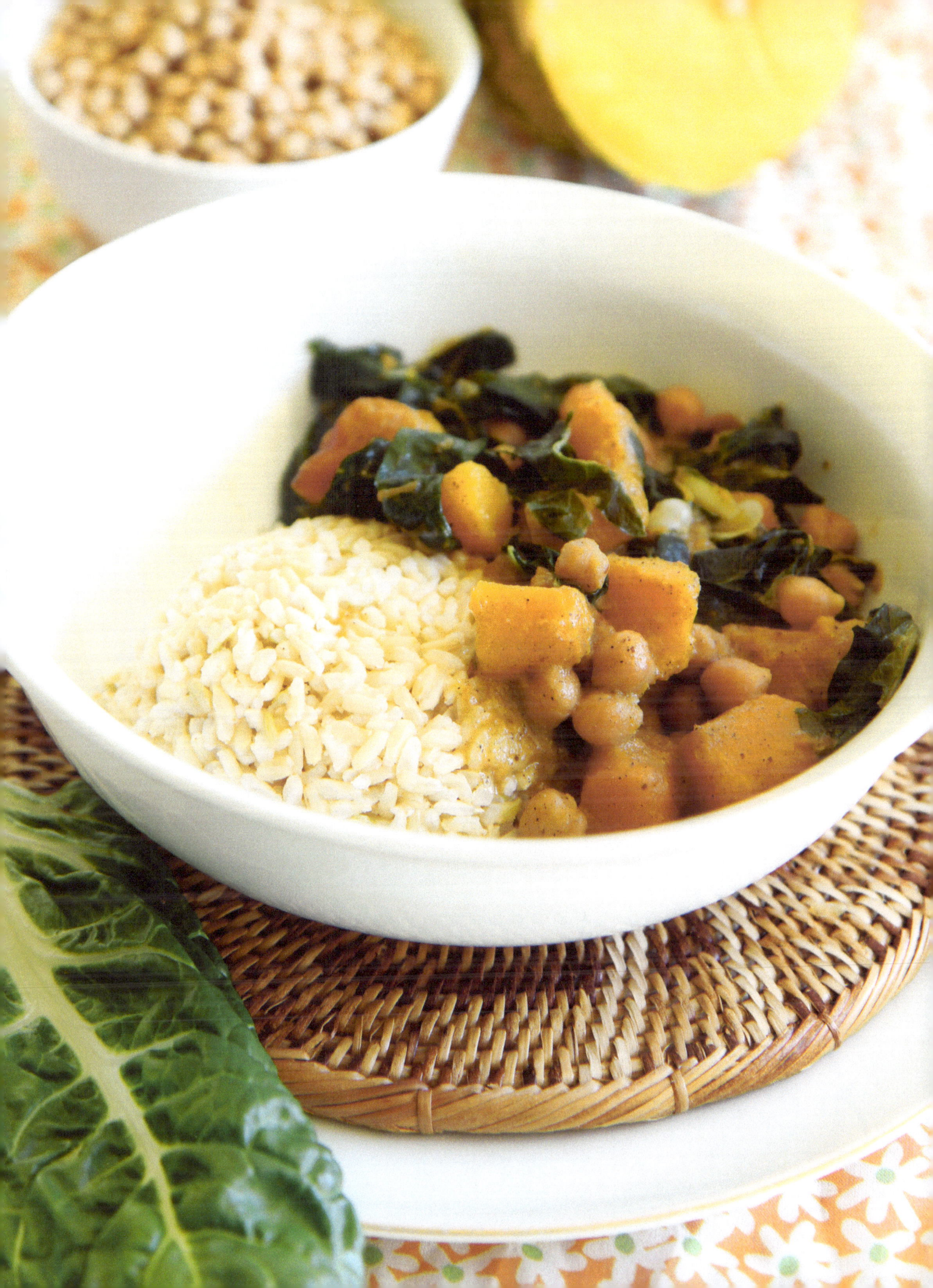

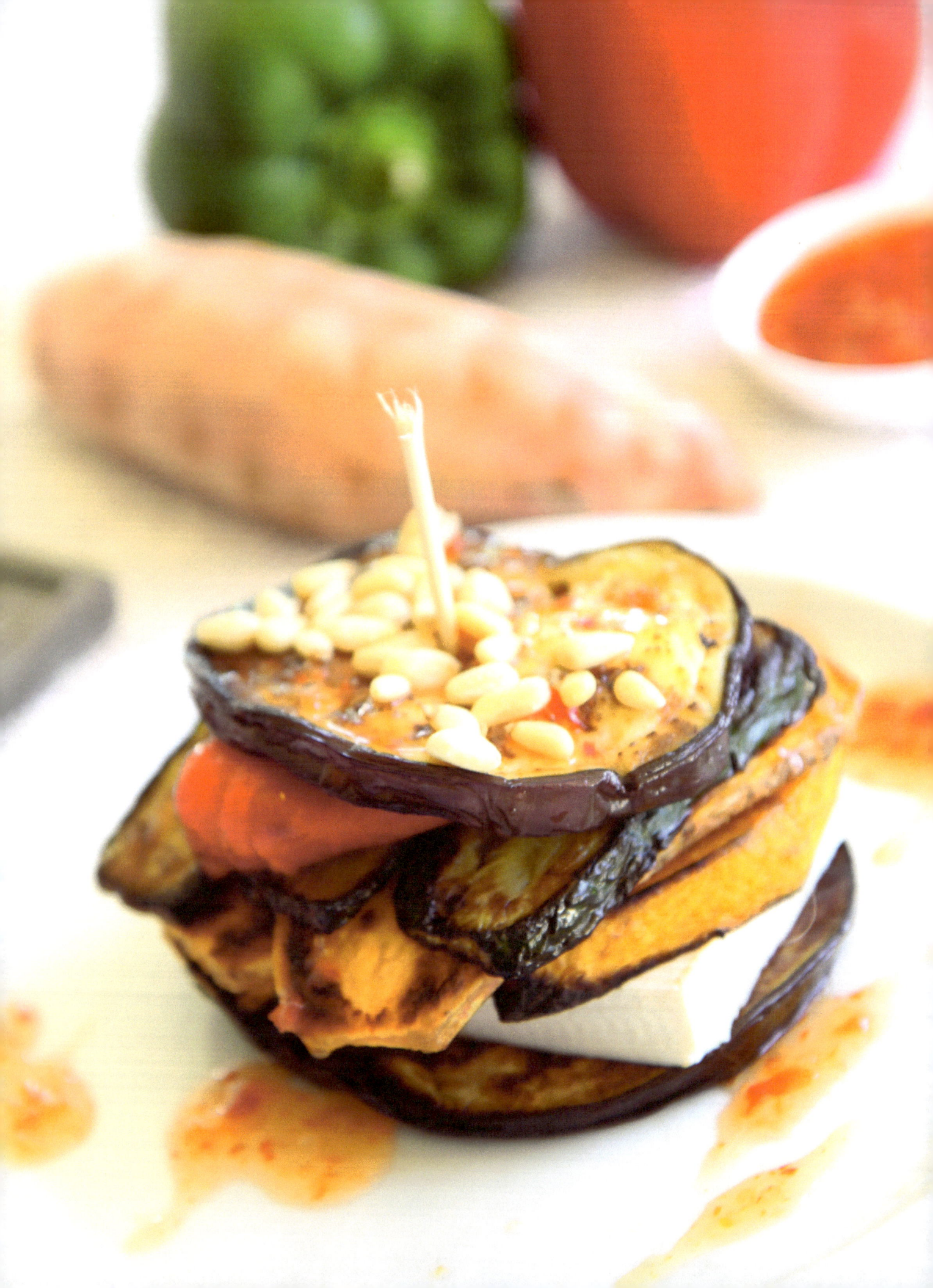

Vegetable Stack

Serves 4 people GF

INGREDIENTS

300g firm tofu, thinly sliced square pieces
1 eggplant (aubergine), thinly sliced
2 zucchinis (courgette), thinly sliced lengthways
1 sweet potato, sliced lengthways
1 red capsicum (pepper), cut into thirds
1 green capsicum (pepper), cut into thirds
¼ pumpkin, sliced
Pine nuts
Sweet chilli sauce
4 bamboo skewers
Extra virgin olive oil

METHOD

- Preheat oven to 180°C (350°F)
- Brush all vegetables with extra virgin olive oil and grill each lot of vegetables separately until cooked, remember to turn onto the other side
- Place grilled capsicum in a plastic bag to help remove the skin, leave for 5-10 minutes and peel off skins
- Let all vegetables cool
- Place on a greased tray 4 slices of eggplant, spread on sweet chilli sauce and sprinkle some pine nuts on top
- Add slice of tofu, then pumpkin, green capsicum, sweet potato, zucchini, red capsicum
- Finish with eggplant on top, spread with some sweet chilli sauce and sprinkle with pine nuts
- Pierce bamboo skewers through the stacks to keep in place
- Cook on medium heat 180°C (350°F) for 30 minutes
- Remove skewers before serving - or not

Note: See who can eat their stack without the pieces falling down

Non-violence leads to the highest ethics, which is the goal of all evolution. Until we stop harming all other living beings, we are still savages.
- Thomas Edison

tempeh satay with asian greens

Serves 2-3 people **GF**

INGREDIENTS

200g tempeh, cut into thin slices
2 bunches of Chinese greens eg Bok choy, chopped
2 cups of broccoli florets
1 zucchini (courgette), thinly sliced
2 tomatoes, diced
1 onion, diced
2 garlic cloves, crushed
¼ cup soymilk
4 tbsp (crunchy) peanut butter
Extra virgin olive oil

METHOD

- Sauté garlic and onion in olive oil in wok
- Add zucchini and broccoli, stir-fry
- Mix in soymilk and peanut butter thoroughly
- Add the tomatoes, tempeh and Chinese greens
- Stir-fry until all ingredients are cooked
- Serve with rice

Awareness is bad for the meat business. Conscience is bad for the meat business. Sensitivity to life is bad for the meat business. DENIAL, however, the meat business finds indispensable.
– John Robbins

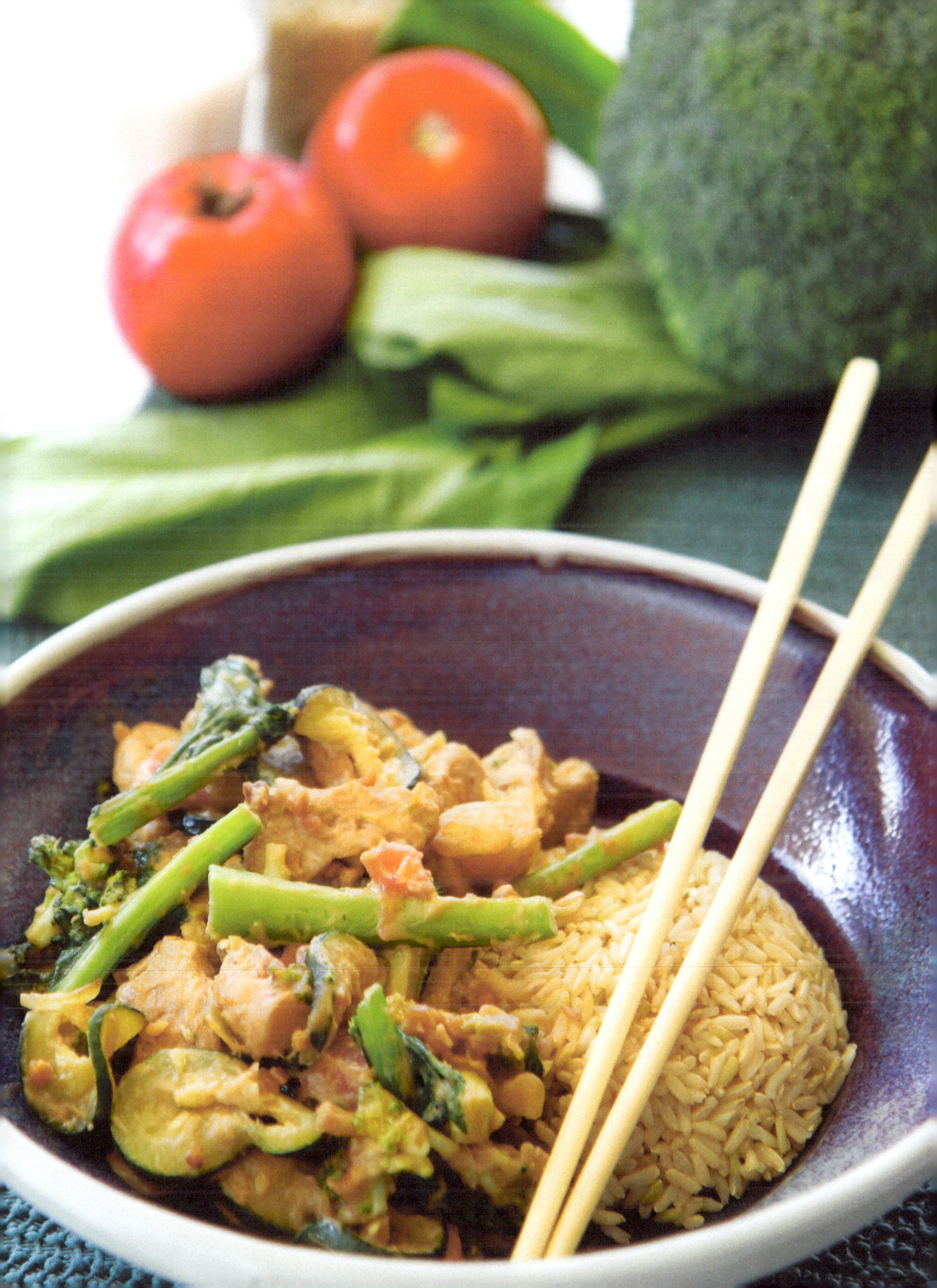

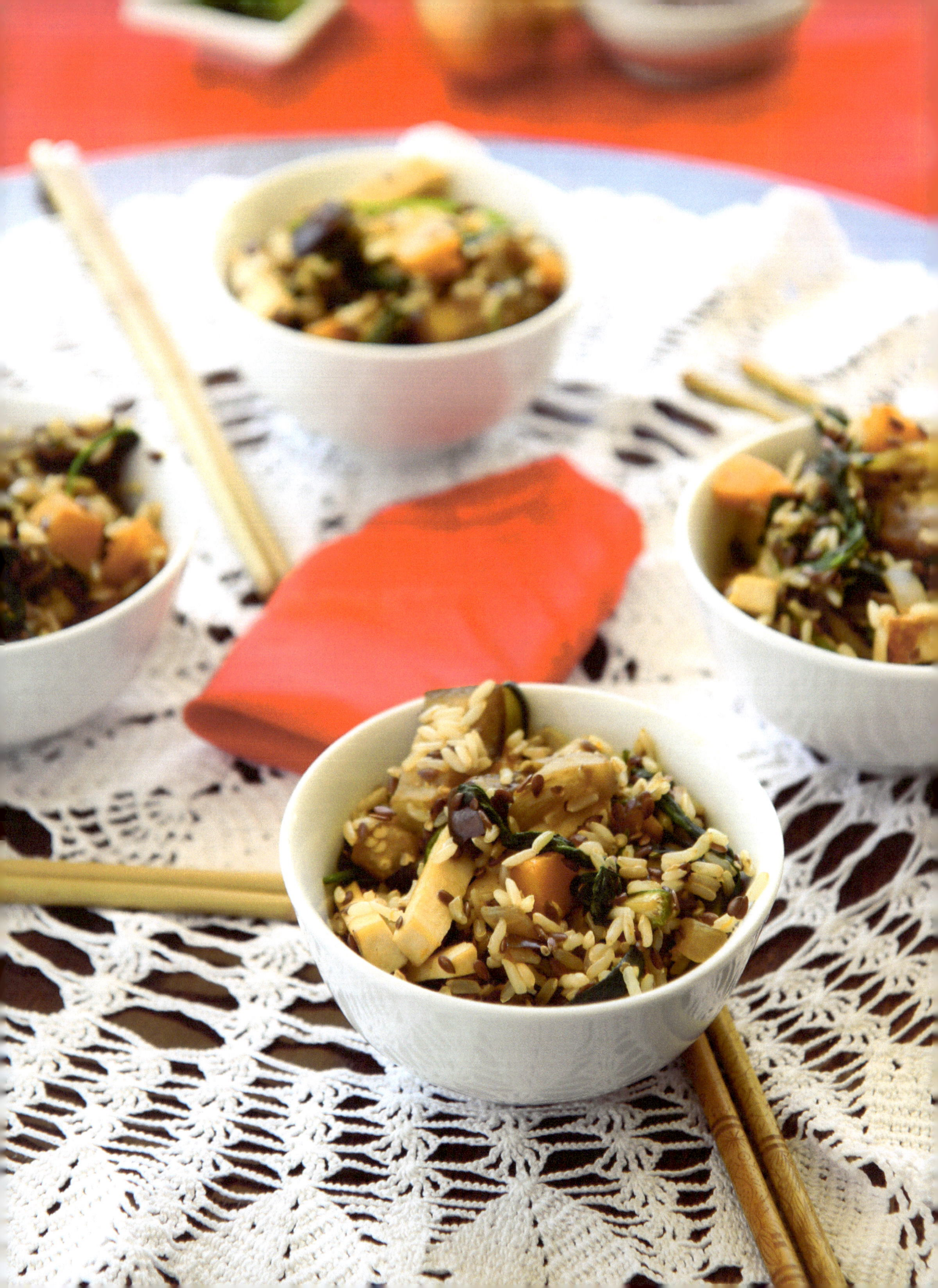

tofu and rice stir-fry

Serves 3-4 people **GF**

INGREDIENTS

300g tofu, cut into large strips
2 cups of brown rice
6 cups of filtered water
1 zucchini (courgette), thinly sliced lengthwise
8 okras, thinly sliced
¼ pumpkin, diced
½ eggplant (aubergine), thinly sliced
½ cup of linseeds
2 handfuls of baby spinach
1 onion, diced
2 garlic cloves, crushed
Extra virgin olive oil

METHOD

- Sauté garlic and onion with oil in wok
- Add pumpkin, zucchini, okra and eggplant; stir-fry until cooked
- Mix through linseeds, tofu, baby spinach and cooked rice
- Serve with seasoned seaweed

Vegetarianism isn't about fanatical personal purity; it's about having some perspective. Move at your own pace; no one's keeping score. Vegetarianism isn't about scarcity; it's about abundance. It's not about restriction; it's about liberation. Not about what we're against but what we're for. Not for some far-off time but for right now. For me going vegetarian is less about becoming something and more about being true to ourselves.

- Michael Gregor MD

ingredients list

Garlic cloves 22, 24, 32, 34, 36, 38, 40, 42, 44, 46, 52, 54, 58, 60, 62, 68, 82, 84, 90, 92

Ginger 24, 32, 38, 54

Gnocchi 52

Hokkein noodles 42

Hummus 66

Lemon – juice, rind and flesh 22

Lemongrass 26

Lentils 26, 40

Linseeds 92

LSA mix (linseed, sunflower and almond) 58, 66, 84

Millet 38, 58

Mung Bean Fettuccine 84

Mushrooms – field 22, 32, 34

Nectarines 30

Nutritional Yeast 60, 72, 84

Okra 38, 52, 92

Olives – kalamata 68

Onion 24, 26, 32, 34, 40, 42, 58, 60, 62, 82, 90, 92

Oregano 30, 44, 60, 82, 84

Parsley 22

Peanut butter – crunchy 90

Peri Peri 34, 40

Pine nuts 56, 70, 88

Pizza bases - gluten free 44

Polenta (corn meal/semolina) 62

Potato 34

Pumpkin 22, 24, 26, 28, 32, 34, 40, 50, 56, 58, 60, 70, 72, 76, 78, 80, 82, 86, 88, 92

Quinoa – white and red 30, 46, 56, 64, 78

Red Kidney beans 24, 36, 76, 78, 82

Rice and Corn Lasagne sheets 60

Rice flakes – thick (Indian) 26

Snow peas (sugar snaps) 56

Soy/vegan cream cheese 36, 44, 72, 76

Soymilk 62, 74, 90

Soy sauce or Tamari 32

Spinach (silverbeet) & baby spinach leaves 36, 38, 40, 42, 52, 60, 62, 84, 86, 92

Squash (marrows) 26, 28, 46, 50, 74, 82

Sun-dried tomatoes or semi dried tomatoes 44, 68

Sweet chilli sauce 34, 42, 80, 88

Sweet Potato (Kumara, similar to a Yam) – orange and purple 22, 24, 26, 34, 50, 72, 74, 80, 86, 88

Tahini (sesame seed paste) – unhulled 28, 44

Tempeh 38, 74, 90

Tofu – firm and silken (soft) 32, 42, 52, 68, 70, 88, 92

Tomatoes 30, 48, 52, 60, 62, 82, 84, 90

Turnip (swede, rutabaga) 26

TVP (Textured Vegetable Protein) or vegan casserole mince 34

Vegan/Soy margarine or butter 22

Vinegar 22

Walnuts 62

Wild rice 48, 68, 82

Zucchini (courgette) 22, 24, 28, 30, 32, 34, 36, 38, 46, 50, 58, 62, 64, 68, 76, 78, 80, 84, 88, 90, 92

Viva la Vegan!

Viva la Vegan! started to promote Leigh-Chantelle's Recipe Calendars in 2005 and has since grown to be an interactive community for vegans, focusing on positive education, information and vegan outreach. Through the vivalavegan.net website, Leigh-Chantelle's focus is on educating people about alternative lifestyle choices, proving that through compassion we can heal ourselves and each other.

Vivalavegan.net focuses on easy-to-prepare recipes, blogs, articles, podcasts, interactive forum, informative and how-to videos, interviews with inspiring vegans, vegan mentoring, eBooks, print books and much more.

You can find Leigh-Chantelle and Viva la Vegan! on:

facebook. g+ 🍎 iTunes Pinterest twitter YouTube

vivalavegan.net

About the author

Leigh-Chantelle is a published author, international speaker and blogger who lives mostly in Brisbane, Australia where she runs the online vegan community Viva la Vegan! and the not-for-profit environmental awareness Green Earth Group. She also coordinates in-person and online coaching for Online Etiquette Education, Engaging Volunteers, Staging Effective Events, Effective Activism and Empowering Vegans.

Leigh-Chantelle is an accredited naturopath, nutritionist and Western herbalist who combines her passion for vegan health along with her natural therapies and healing skills. She has released three Viva la Vegan! recipe calendars, a plant-based Detox Diet eBook, various other recipe eBooks, re-released her recipe calendars as recycled recipe cards and has published many other print books.

Over the past 16 years since Leigh-Chantelle has been a vegan, she has been involved as a sponsor, performer, speaker, MC and stallholder for various animal rights, vegan, vegetarian, environmental and cruelty-free fundraisers, forums, conferences, festivals and events throughout Australia and Internationally.

Leigh-Chantelle is available for select speaking engagements, seminars, panel discussions and readings on the following:

- Veganism, Animal Rights and Activism
- Staging Effective Events, Engaging Volunteers and Team Work
- Online Etiquette, Social Media Marketing and Online Skills

To enquire about a possible appearance, please contact email@leigh-chantelle.com

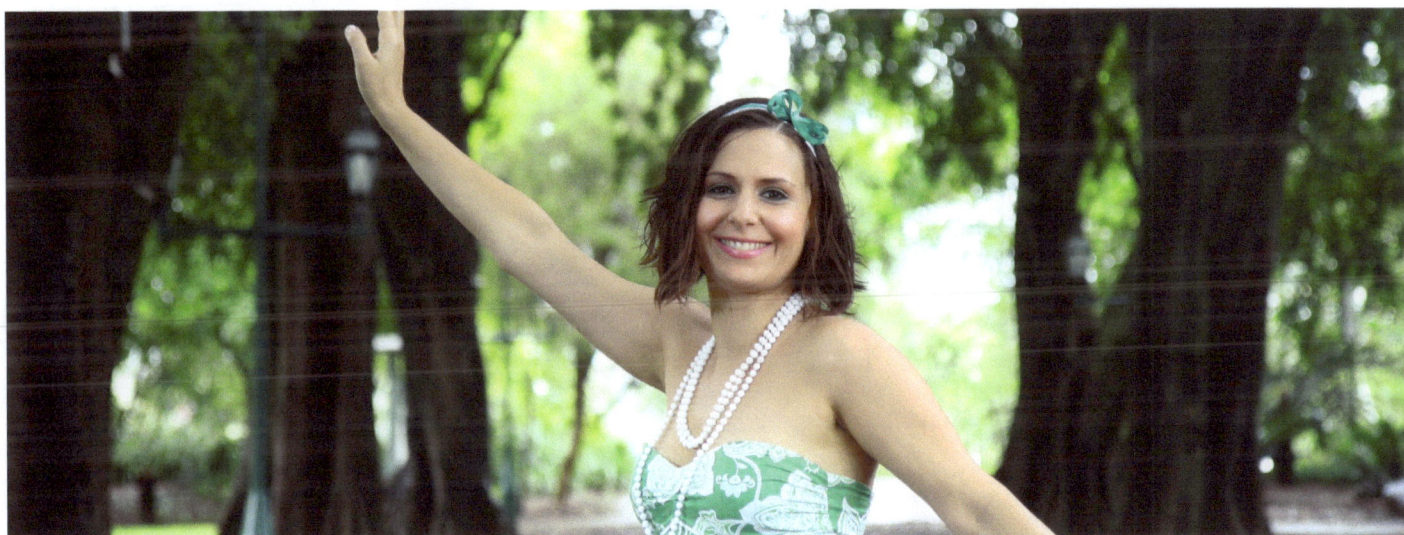

Photo by Carol Slater

About the Photographer

Carol Slater became a full-time photographer after finishing her studies in 2004. Weddings, portraits, music and events have kept her very busy over the last few years. A vegetarian for over 20 years and vegan for 4 years, Carol offers her photography skills to help give a voice to the billions of animals who are exploited in the name of food, fashion, entertainment and research. Carol works with various animal rights and rescue groups in Brisbane, Australia and her images are often seen in magazines, brochures and online.

See Carol's website c-s-p.com.au

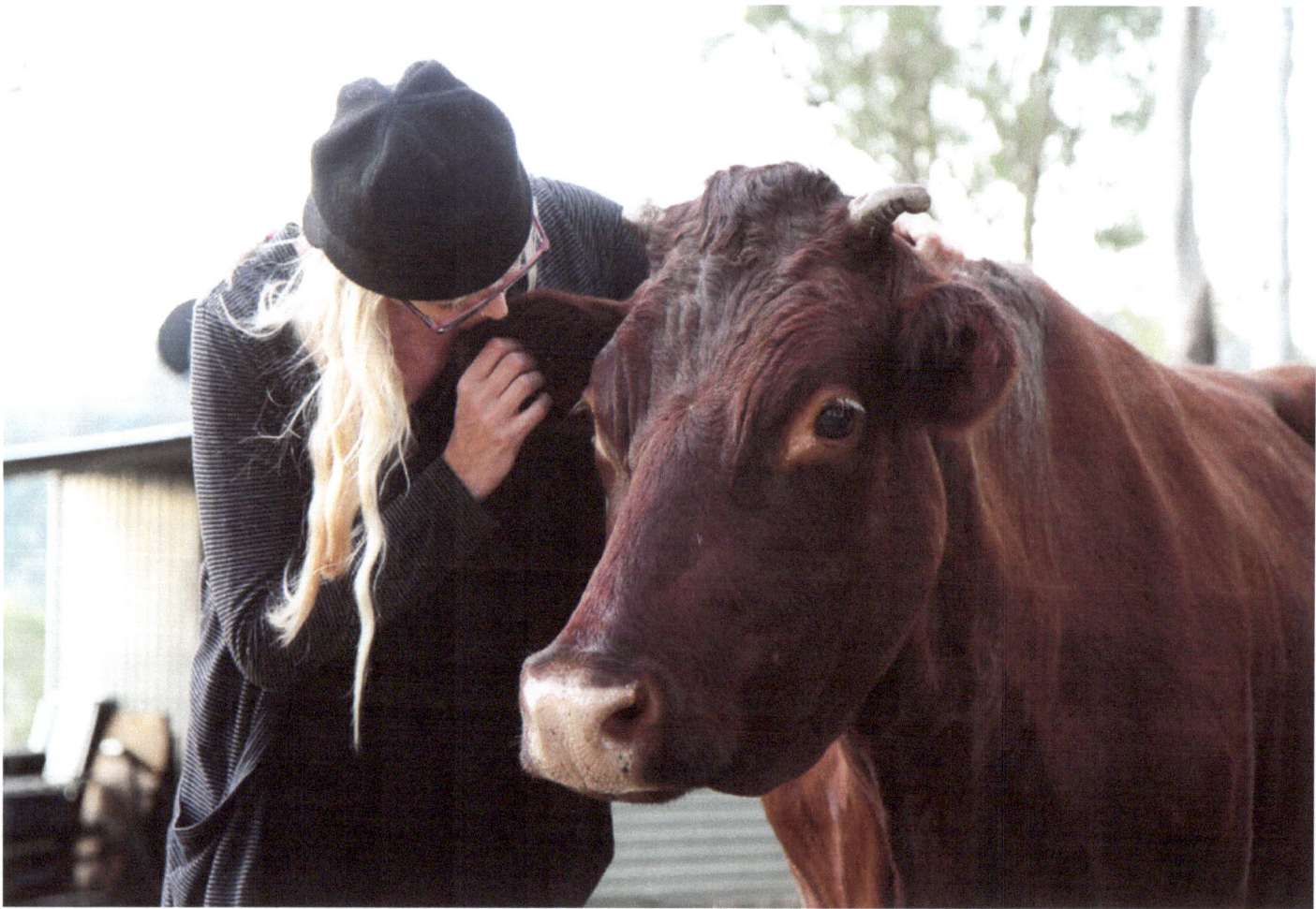

Photo by Natasha Fox

About the Illustrator

Sarah Kiser is a full-time, self-taught artist living her dream of creating art. Infusing layers of richly textured colour with elements of whimsy, her artwork presents imagery that is at once hauntingly beautiful yet fiercely evocative - touching the viewer in a deeply personal way. A vegetarian since childhood, Sarah became a vegan and animal rights activist when she uncovered the cruelty behind the dairy and egg industries. She bases much of her artwork on animals and animal rights, hoping to inspire compassion in those who see her artwork. Sarah is a mother of two boys and lives in Florida, USA. Some of her inspirations are Matisse, Chagall, Van Gogh, Gaughuin, Klmit, and Frida Kahlo.

You can purchase Sarah's artwork and find out more information on her website artbysarahkiser.com

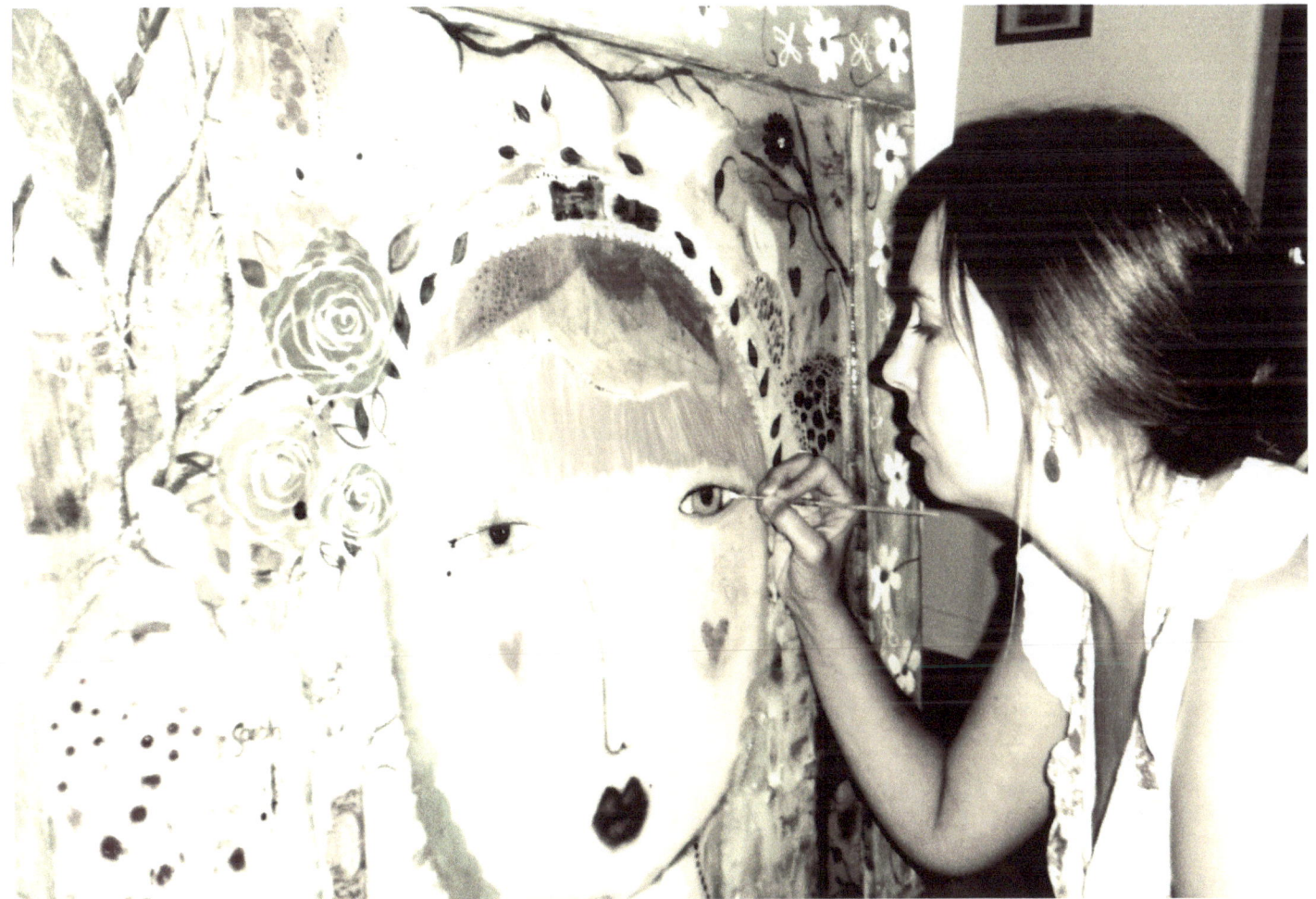

Photo by Christopher Kiser

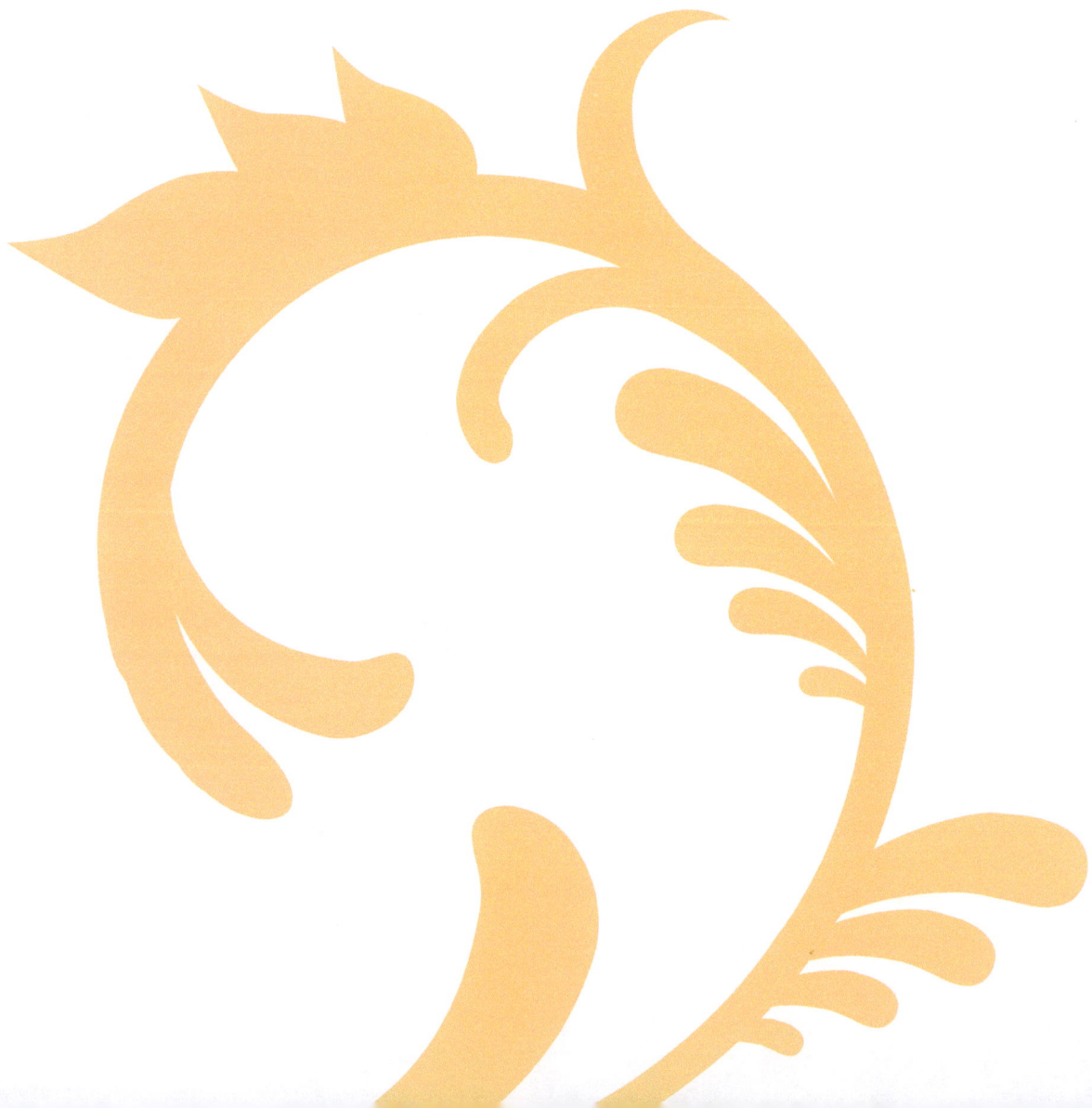

Other Books by Leigh-Chantelle

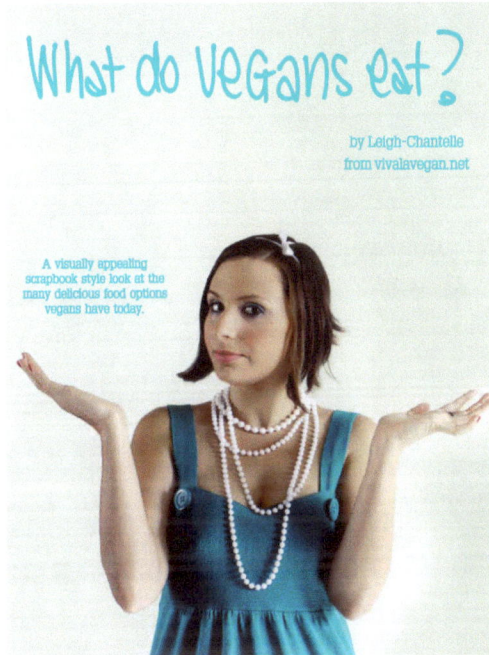

What Do Vegans Eat?

ISBN 978-0-9808484-0-3

Digtial ISBN 978-0-9808484-1-0

2012

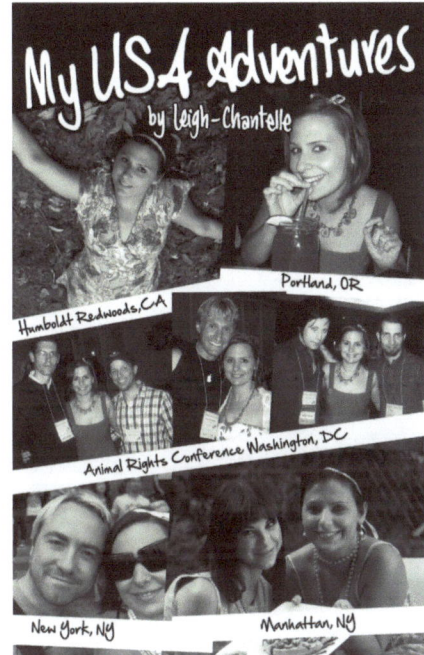

My USA Adventures

ISBN 978-0-9808484-2-7

Digital ISBN 978-0-9808484-3-4

2012

eBooks

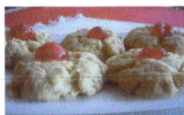
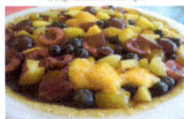
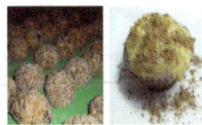
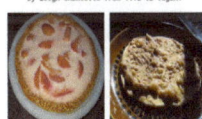
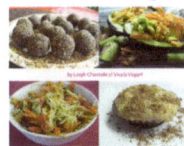
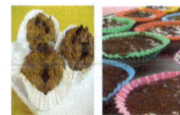
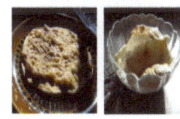
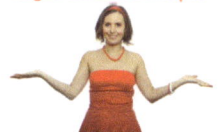

vivalavegan.net/community/store.html

www.ingramcontent.com/pod-product-compliance
Lightning Source LLC
Chambersburg PA
CBHW041955100426
42812CB00018B/2661